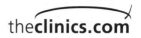

theclinics.com

ANESTHESIOLOGY CLINICS OF NORTH AMERICA

Obesity and Sleep Apnea

GUEST EDITOR
Peter Rock, MD, MBA, FCCP, FCCM

CONSULTING EDITOR
Lee A. Fleisher, MD

September 2005 • Volume 23 • Number 3

SAUNDERS

An Imprint of Elsevier, Inc.
PHILADELPHIA   LONDON   TORONTO   MONTREAL   SYDNEY   TO

W.B. SAUNDERS COMPANY
A Division of Elsevier Inc.

1600 John F. Kennedy Boulevard, Suite 1800 • Philadelphia, Pennsylvania 19103-2899

http://www.theclinics.com

ANESTHESIOLOGY CLINICS OF NORTH AMERICA	Volume 23, Number 3
September 2005	ISSN 0889-8537
Editor: Rachel Glover	ISBN 1-4160-2808-0

The ideas and opinions expressed in *Anesthesiology Clinics of North America* do not necessarily reflect those of the Publisher. The Publisher does not assume any responsibility for any injury and/or damage to persons or property arising out of or related to any use of the material contained in this periodical. The reader is advised to check the appropriate medical literature and the product information currently provided by the manufacturer of each drug to be administered to verify the dosage, the method and duration of administration, or contraindications. It is the responsibility of the treating physician or other health care professional, relying on independent experience and knowledge of the patient, to determine drug dosages and the best treatment for the patient. Mention of any product in this issue should not be construed as endorsement by the contributors, editors, or the Publisher of the product or manufacturers' claims.

Anesthesiology Clinics of North America (ISSN 0889-8537) is published quarterly by the W.B. Saunders Company Corporate and editorial offices: 1600 John F. Kennedy Boulevard, Suite 1800, Philadelphia, PA 19103-2899. Accounting and circulation offices: 6277 Sea Harbor Drive, Orlando, FL 32887-4800. Periodicals postage paid at Orlando, FL 32862, and additional mailing offices. Subscription prices are $84.00 per year (US student/resident), $175.00 per year (US individuals), $210.00 per year (Canadian individuals), $270.00 per year (US institutions), $330.00 per year (Canadian institutions), $230.00 per year (foreign individuals), and $330.00 per year (foreign institutions). To receive student and resident rate, orders must be accompanied by name of affiliated institution, date of term, and the *signature* of program/residency coordinator on institutions letterhead. Orders will be billed at individual rate until proof of status is received. Foreign air speed delivery is included in all *Clinics'* subscription prices. All prices are subject to change without notice. POSTMASTER: Send address changes to *Anesthesiology Clinics of North America*, W.B. Saunders Company, Periodicals Fullfillment, Orlando, FL 32887-4800. Customer Service: 1-800-654-2452 (US). From outside of the US, call 1-407-345-4000. E-mail: hhspcs@wbsaunders.com.

Anesthesiology Clinics of North America is also published in Spanish by McGraw-Hill Interamericana Editores S. A., P.O. Box 5-237, 06500 Mexico D. F., Mexico.

Anesthesiology Clinics of North America is covered in *Index Medicus, Current Contents/Clinical Medicine, Excerpta Medica, ISI/BIOMED,* and *Chemical Abstracts.*

Printed in the United States of America.

CONSULTING EDITOR

LEE A. FLEISHER, MD, Robert D. Dripps Professor and Chair, Departments of Anesthesiology and Critical Care and Medicine, University of Pennsylvania School of Medicine, Philadelphia, Pennsylvania

GUEST EDITOR

PETER ROCK, MD, MBA, FCCP, FCCM, Professor of Anesthesiology and Medicine, Vice-Chair, Department of Anesthesiology, University of North Carolina School of Medicine, Chapel Hill, North Carolina

CONTRIBUTORS

PREETAM BANDLA, MD, Fellow, Pulmonary Medicine, Pulmonary Division, Sleep Disorders Center, Children's Hospital of Philadelphia; University of Pennsylvania School of Medicine, Philadelphia, Pennsylvania

ROBERT L. BELL, MD, MA, Assistant Professor, Department of Surgery, Yale University School of Medicine, New Haven, Connecticut

LEE J. BROOKS, MD, Pulmonary Division, Sleep Disorders Center, Children's Hospital of Philadelphia; Clinical Associate Professor of Pediatrics, University of Pennsylvania School of Medicine, Philadelphia, Pennsylvania

RAFAEL CARTAGENA, MD, Assistant Professor, Department of Anesthesiology, University of North Carolina School of Medicine, Chapel Hill, North Carolina

MARION EVERETT COUCH, MD, PhD, Assistant Professor, Department of Otolaryngology–Head and Neck Surgery, University of North Carolina School of Medicine, Chapel Hill, North Carolina

EUGENE B. FREID, MD, FCCM, Department of Anesthesiology, Nemours Children's Clinics, Jacksonville, Florida; Professor of Anesthesiology and Pediatrics; Medical Director, Respiratory Care; Departments of Anesthesiology and Pediatrics, University of North Carolina School of Medicine, Chapel Hill, North Carolina

MARK HELFAER, MD, FCCM, Professor of Anesthesiology and Pediatrics, University of Pennsylvania School of Medicine; Endowed Chair and Chief, Critical Care Medicine, Children's Hospital of Philadelphia, Philadelphia, Pennsylvania

KENNETH F. KUCHTA, MD, Assistant Clinical Professor, Department of Anesthesiology, David Geffen School of Medicine at UCLA, Los Angeles, California

PATRICK J. NELIGAN, MD, Assistant Professor, Department of Anesthesia, University of Pennsylvania School of Medicine, Philadelphia, Pennsylvania

ANNETTE G. PASHAYAN, MD, Associate Professor of Anesthesiology, Department of Anesthesiology, University of North Carolina School of Medicine, Chapel Hill, North Carolina

ANTHONY N. PASSANNANTE, MD, Associate Professor of Anesthesiology, Department of Anesthesiology, University of North Carolina School of Medicine, Chapel Hill, North Carolina

SUSAN L. POLK, MD, MSEd, Professor of Clinical Anesthesia and Critical Care Medicine, Pritzker School of Medicine, University of Chicago, Chicago, Illinois

NARESH M. PUNJABI, MD, PhD, Department of Medicine, Johns Hopkins University School of Medicine, Baltimore, Maryland

PETER ROCK, MD, MBA, FCCP, FCCM, Professor of Anesthesiology and Medicine, Vice-Chair, Department of Anesthesiology, University of North Carolina School of Medicine, Chapel Hill, North Carolina

STANLEY H. ROSENBAUM, MD, Professor of Anesthesiology, Internal Medicine, and Surgery, Department of Anesthesiology, Yale University School of Medicine; Private Practice, New Haven, Connecticut

BRENT SENIOR, MD, Associate Professor, Department of Otolaryngology–Head and Neck Surgery, University of North Carolina School of Medicine, Chapel Hill, North Carolina

TRACEY STIERER, MD, Department of Anesthesiology and Critical Care Medicine, Johns Hopkins University School of Medicine, Baltimore, Maryland

TARA TRIMARCHI, MSN, RN, Pediatric Intensive Care Unit, Children's Hospital of Philadelphia, Philadelphia, Pennsylvania

AVERY TUNG, MD, Associate Professor, Department of Anesthesia and Critical Care, University of Chicago, Chicago, Illinois

NOËL WILLIAMS, MD, Director, Bariatric Surgery Program, Department of Surgery, University of Pennsylvania School of Medicine, Philadelphia, Pennsylvania

CONTENTS

The incidence of obesity is increasing yearly among adults and children in the United States and worldwide. Although there is a significant genetic component to obesity, the genome has not changed. The epidemic is caused by an increase in dietary fat and caloric input and a decrease in physical activity. There are significant racial, ethnic, and sociologic differences in all categories of obesity as well as in the disease burden it brings. The effects of the obesity epidemic are considerable, second only to tobacco use in the expenditure of health care dollars and as a cause of premature mortality.

This article reviews the terminology of obstructive sleep apnea and the associated diagnostic tests and provides an overview of the risk factors for this chronic condition. Sleep apnea affects 2% to 4% of middle-aged working adults in the general population, however, a considerable number of affected individuals remain undiagnosed. Patients with the disease may be at a higher risk for adverse perioperative outcomes. Knowledge of factors associated with an increased risk of obstructive sleep apnea is vital to the perioperative assessment and anesthetic plan.

FORTHCOMING ISSUES

December 2005

March 2006

June 2006

RECENT ISSUES

June 2005

March 2005

December 2004

THE CLINICS ARE NOW AVAILABLE ONLINE!

For more information about Clinics:
http://www.theclinics.com

ELSEVIER
SAUNDERS

Anesthesiology Clin N Am
23 (2005) xi–xii

ANESTHESIOLOGY
CLINICS OF
NORTH AMERICA

Foreword

Obesity and Sleep Apnea

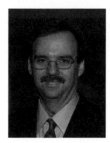

Lee A. Fleisher, MD
Consulting Editor

Obesity is clearly becoming one of the most common medical comorbidities seen by the practicing anesthesiologist. In addition to affecting virtually every major organ system, it is frequently associated with obstructive sleep apnea. It is becoming evident to most practitioners that obstructive sleep apnea occurs much more frequently in clinical practice than formally diagnosed, and that this condition represents complex challenges for clinical care and decisions regarding postoperative monitoring and discharge status. In this issue of the *Anesthesiology Clinics of North America*, an excellent group of leaders in the field have contributed articles on issues of pathophysiology and practice management of this group of patients.

We are fortunate to have Peter Rock as the Guest Editor for this issue. Peter is currently Professor of Anesthesiology and Medicine at the University of North Carolina at Chapel Hill and Vice-Chair of the Department of Anesthesiology. He is also the Medical Director of the Preoperative Evaluation Clinic, the Intermediate Surgical Care Unit, the Division of Critical Care Medicine, and Associate Director of the Operating Rooms. He has published 56 original articles and 33 book chapters, and this represents the second issue of the *Anesthesiology Clinics of North America* he has edited in the past 5 years. His background and

0889-8537/05/$ – see front matter © 2005 Elsevier Inc. All rights reserved.
doi:10.1016/j.atc.2005.06.001   *anesthesiology.theclinics.com*

current responsibilities make him the ideal individual to assemble an issue that focuses on this complex and timely topic.

Lee A. Fleisher, MD
Departments of Anesthesiology and Critical Care and Medicine
University of Pennsylvania School of Medicine
3400 Spruce Street, Dulles 690
Philadelphia, PA 19104, USA
E-mail address: fleishel@uphs.upenn.edu

Anesthesiology Clin N Am
23 (2005) xiii–xv

ANESTHESIOLOGY
CLINICS OF
NORTH AMERICA

Preface

Obesity and Sleep Apnea

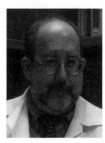

Peter Rock, MD, MBA, FCCP, FCCM
Guest Editor

Obesity in America has been referred to as a new epidemic. Its incidence is increasing, as are the number of patients that are morbidly obese. Obstructive sleep apnea (OSA) also is being recognized and diagnosed with increasing frequency. In some subsets of the population, OSA is as prevalent as a chronic disease such as asthma. Obesity is a risk factor for OSA. These two conditions, obesity and OSA, pose significant challenges for anesthesiologists and other health care providers engaged in the care of surgical patients. This issue of the *Anesthesiology Clinics of North America* is devoted to aspects of perioperative care of individuals with obesity and OSA.

In "Definitions and Demographics of Obesity: Diagnosis and Risk Factors," Susan Polk discusses the epidemiology of obesity. She documents the alarming increase in obesity and morbid obesity as well as interesting geographic associations. There are important racial and ethnic differences in the prevalence of obesity in the United States. The number of children who have obesity is also increasing, and Dr. Polk covers issues related to this disturbing trend. Obesity has important economic and societal implications that are detailed in this article, especially those that impact public health. Drs. Stierer and Punjabi comprehensively review the "Demographics and Diagnosis of Obstructive Sleep Apnea." This article saliently reviews terminology used in individuals with OSA as well as diagnostic tests and results that may be encountered when caring for patients who have this disorder. The prevalence of OSA is described, including insight into how the definition of diagnostic abnormalities influences the incidence of disease. Risk factors for OSA are described which are important as the perioperative caregiver may be the first to suspect or even diagnose the presence of OSA. Understanding risk factors for OSA is the first step in diagnosis.

Ken Kuchta reviews the "Pathophysiologic Changes of Obesity." In this article, the effect of obesity on cardiovascular disease is documented. Kuchta carefully reviews the metabolic syndrome: an important new concept relating obesity, dyslipidemia, hypertension and impaired glucose regulation. The role of leptin in obesity and mediators linked to adipose tissue are also reviewed. Obesity can significantly impact the respiratory system, which is covered here as well. The "Pathophysiology of Obstructive Sleep Apnea" is covered by Pashayan, Passannante, and Rock. In this review, the authors describe the location and cause of airway obstruction. Important nonanatomic contributors to OSA are also reviewed. Signs and symptoms of OSA are categorized. There are other diseases associated with OSA, and their recognition is important, because they may be the first clue to the presence of OSA.

Avery Tung reviews the "Biology and Genetics of Obesity and Obstructive Sleep Apnea." As might be expected, there is a wealth of emerging information about the biology of these disorders. Genetic variability appears to play a key role in the development of OSA. Understanding genetic factors might allow improved screening for the disease as well as identify factors that result in either worse or better outcomes after surgery. The genetic interaction between obesity and OSA is also reviewed with emphasis on craniofacial abnormalities, ventilatory control, and sleep regulation. The "Preoperative Evaluation of Patients with Obesity and Obstructive Sleep Apnea" is reviewed by Rafael Cartagena. Risk assessment in these populations is reviewed. Clearly, airway assessment is especially important in these populations and is covered in detail. Cardiopulmonary assessment is also reviewed in the setting of obesity and OSA. Identification of the patient at risk for OSA is reviewed, as are interventions and treatments that may reduce risk in these patients.

The "Anesthetic Management of Patients with Obesity and Sleep Apnea" is covered by Passannante and Rock. The authors review the pharmacokinetics of drugs in obese patients. Positioning obese patients may be problematic and may lead to complications, and this topic is reviewed in detail. Regional anesthesia and monitoring needs for obese patients are also covered. Patients with OSA have unique anesthetic considerations covered in this section as well, such as the effect of anesthetic drugs on ventilatory responses and type of appropriate monitoring. Bell and Rosenbaum review "Postoperative Considerations for Patients with Obesity and Sleep Apnea." Individuals who have these conditions require special care after surgery, and the authors review the implications of obesity and OSA for the postoperative period. The important issue of postoperative monitoring and the need for special observation is discussed. Pain management takes on additional importance in these patients, and the authors detail special considerations for analgesia under these conditions.

Because obese patients may present to the operating room for surgery to treat their obesity, it is important to understand these procedures. Drs. Neligan and Williams review "Nonsurgical and Surgical Treatment of Obesity." Nonsurgical management of obesity is reviewed, including pharmacologic measures that have anesthetic implications. Surgical treatment measures are covered in detail. Perioperative management of individuals undergoing bariatric surgery is comprehensively reviewed. Outcomes, complications, and long-term follow-up after obesity surgery are covered as well. The article concludes with the future of treatments for obesity. Given the increased occurrence of OSA in the population, and its significant impact on health, treatment of this condition has become increasingly important, covered by Drs. Couch and Senior in "Nonsurgical and Surgical Treatments for Sleep Apnea." Medical management of OSA is reviewed, including positive airway pressure and oral appliances. Surgical treatment options are discussed. New advances in minimally invasive procedures are discussed, as are future areas of research and possible treatments. The article concludes with a review of perioperative issues specific to OSA surgery.

Children may develop OSA and are a special group of patients. Bandla, Brooks, Trimarchi, and Helfaer review "Obstructive Sleep Apnea Syndrome in Children." The differences between the presentation, pathophysiology, and treatment in adults and children are documented. Perioperative management considerations in children with OSA are reviewed, as are anesthetic considerations. Postoperative care issues are covered in detail, as is pain management in this special group of patients. Finally, the natural history and prognosis of children with OSA is discussed.

Our final article covers "The Rapid Sequence Induction Revisited: The Obese Patient and Sleep Apnea Syndrome," authored by Eugene Fried. Obese patients may be considered at risk for pulmonary aspiration of gastric contents, thus rapid sequence induction may be employed in these patients. Whether these patients really are at increased risk is discussed, as are the benefits and potential risks of rapid sequence induction and application of cricoid pressure. The evidence underlying the effectiveness of these maneuvers is also reviewed.

This issue of the *Anesthesiology Clinics of North America* comprehensively covers a variety of topics relevant to the perioperative management of patients with obesity and OSA. It should prove a valuable resource for those who care for such patients.

Peter Rock, MD, MBA, FCCP, FCCM
Department of Anesthesiology
University of North Carolina School of Medicine
N2201, CB# 7010
Chapel Hill, NC 27599-7010, USA
E-mail address: prock@aims.unc.edu

ELSEVIER
SAUNDERS

Anesthesiology Clin N Am
23 (2005) 397–403

ANESTHESIOLOGY
CLINICS OF
NORTH AMERICA

Definitions and Demographics of Obesity: Diagnosis and Risk Factors

Susan L. Polk, MD, MSEd

*Pritzker School of Medicine, University of Chicago, 5841 South Maryland Avenue, Box MC4028,
Chicago, IL 60637, USA*

Obesity is defined by the body mass index (BMI). The BMI is calculated according to the formula weight (kg) divided by height squared (m^2). The normal BMI range is 18.5–25, and the range 25–30 is considered overweight. The National Institutes of Health classifies obesity by degrees [1]: class 1, BMI 30–35; class 2, BMI 35–40; and class 3, BMI greater than 40 (morbid obesity).

The medical and public news has recently been full of alarming stories about the increasing prevalence and consequences of obesity in the United States and worldwide. The World Health Organization describes "globesity" as an epidemic affecting at least 300 million people, with an increase of at least 3-fold since 1980 in parts of Eastern Europe, the Middle East, China, and the Pacific Islands [2]. In 2000, the worldwide number of obese people exceeded the number of underweight people. In 2001, in the United States, the prevalence of obesity (BMI ≥30) was 20.9% [3]. Morbid obesity was present in 2.3% of the population, and the prevalence reaches 67% if the category of overweight is included (BMI ≥25) [4]. The incidence of class 3 obesity increased 3-fold from 1990 to 2000 [5]. Fig. 1 shows obesity trends among US adults by state in 1991, 1996, and 2003 [6]. Mississippi, Alabama, West Virginia, and Indiana showed an obesity rate of 25% or more in 2003; and no state reported a rate less than 15%. States with 15% to 19% were Arizona, Colorado, Connecticut, Florida, Hawaii, Maine, Massachusetts, Montana, New Hampshire, New Jersey, New Mexico, Rhode Island, Utah, Vermont, and Wyoming. Colorado has the lowest historical rate and still does. It is estimated that if current trends continue, 40% of the US population will be obese in 2010 [7].

E-mail address: spolk@dacc.uchicago.edu

0889-8537/05/$ – see front matter © 2005 Elsevier Inc. All rights reserved.
doi:10.1016/j.atc.2005.03.005   *anesthesiology.theclinics.com*

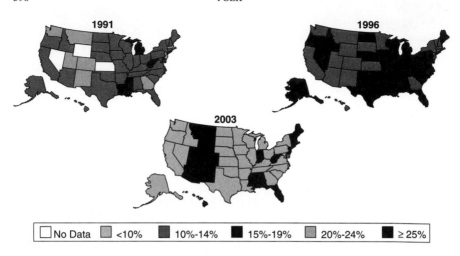

Fig. 1. Obesity trend surveys for 1991, 1996, and 2003 among US adults. Obesity was defined as a BMI greater than 30, or approximately 30 lbs overweight for an individual 5 ft 4 in tall. (*Data from* National Center for Chronic Disease Prevention and Health Promotion. Obesity trends among US adults between 1985 and 2003. Available at: www.cdc.gov/nccdphp/dnpa/obesity/. Accessed December 2, 2004.)

Evidence suggests the prevalence of significant racial and ethnic differences in obesity in the United States, with overrepresentation in the African-American, Latino, and Asian subpopulations. The rate of rise in prevalence is greatest among African-American women, second greatest among Hispanic women, and third greatest among white women [8]. There is little difference in prevalence among ethnic groups of men. Foreign-born immigrants to the United States generally have a lower prevalence of obesity, but this rate approaches that of US natives with longer residence [9].

The incidence of childhood obesity is rising at an alarming rate, and it has been attributed to the same lifestyle factors as adult obesity. The Centers for Disease Control prefers to define childhood overweight as a BMI greater than the 95th percentile, according to growth charts for the United States in 2000. A 2004 fact sheet prepared by the Institute of Medicine [10] noted that the incidence of obesity has doubled for children in the age groups 2 to 5 and 12 to 19 years since 1970, and during that time period, the incidence has tripled for children in the age group 6 to 12 years. The interesting facts in those statistics are that the leanest children are remaining lean as the others gain weight and that the heaviest group of children is getting heavier. These trends are mirrored in the US adult population and worldwide. The epidemic affects both girls and boys and encompasses all ages and race groups. Among boys, the prevalence is highest in Hispanic, American Indian, and African-American groups. Among girls, the highest prevalence is in African Americans. The southern United States show a higher prevalence than the north, and the children of lower socioeconomic status are more at risk than the higher.

Factors implicated in the childhood epidemic include the following:

- Urban and suburban plans that discourage walking and other physical activities
- Increasing consumption of convenience and fast foods that are high in calories and fat
- Expense and lack of access in some communities to fresh fruits and vegetables and other nutritious foods
- Reduced physical activities available during and after school
- Reduced walking or biking to and from school
- Television, computers, and videogames that are replacing outdoor leisure time activities

Obese mothers, especially if they are diabetic, produce children of increased birth weight who are likely to be obese throughout life. Obese children and adolescents have a higher incidence of diabetes mellitus, obstructive sleep apnea, tibia vera, polycystic ovary syndrome, fatty liver disease, hyperinsulinemia, and dyslipidemia, depression, and anxiety than their normal counterparts [11]. They miss more school, and they rate their health-related quality of life lower in all domains (physical, psychosocial, emotional, social, and school functioning). Their self-reported quality of life is as equally impaired as that reported for children and adolescents with cancer and those undergoing chemotherapy.

Although genetics is a factor in excess weight, it is not considered to be a factor in the epidemic, because over the last three decades the genetic makeup of the population has not been considered to have changed appreciably. Twin studies [12,13] indicate that as much as 70% of variability in human weight may be accounted for by genetic factors. Approximately 30 Mendelian disorders have been described, with obesity as one characteristic. In most cases, the defective gene product is an intracellular protein with a whole-body function [14]. Energy expenditure consists of the amount of energy required to maintain homeostasis and metabolize food and the amount expended as a result of activity. The obesity epidemic is directly related to the last of those factors. As of 1998, only 25% of US adults were meeting the current recommendation of 30 minutes of leisure time physical activity on most days [15]. The dietary habits of adults as well as children have become less healthy because of many factors associated with lifestyle. Our lives are increasingly sedentary, and our employment is less physical.

Several genes that participate in body weight have been identified, but monogenetic causes in humans are rare. The first major advance was the discovery of the adipocyte-derived hormone leptin, soon followed by discovery of the leptin receptor in the hypothalamus. Leptin acts apparently to signal adequate energy input and thus moderate appetite in the hypothalamus but also may have peripheral effects. Mutations disrupting the leptin and leptin receptor genes have been discovered in humans, and the chromosomal locus containing the leptin gene has been linked to human obesity [16]. Studies to determine the safety and efficacy of recombinant human leptin are in progress, and results have been encouraging in humans shown to have a genetic deficiency of leptin [14]. Leptin-deficient humans have early-onset obesity, increased food intake, hypogonadotropic hypogonadism, hyperinsulinemia, defective function of the hypothalo-pituitary-thyroidal axis, and defects in T-cell number and function. Heterozygote subjects for the leptin-deficient gene show a partial leptin deficiency and average a mean fat mass 23% greater than predicted by their height and weight [17].

A genetic mutation causing leptin-receptor deficiency has also been discovered in humans, resulting in rapid weight gain in the first few months of life after a normal birth weight. The metabolic rate and cortisol levels were normal, but there was hyperinsulinemia with normoglycemia (insulin resistance) [14]. This genetic mutation, which is well studied in mice [18], does not respond to leptin therapy.

Known secondary messenger systems in the hypothalamus include neurons expressing neuropeptide Y and agouti-related peptide, which are suppressed by leptin administration, and neurons expressing the products of pro-opiomelano-cortin (POMC), which are stimulated by leptin administration [18]. POMC is cleaved into α melanocyte-stimulating hormone and adrenocorticotropic hormone. Mutations in the POMC gene sequence are associated with a syndrome of obesity, red hair, and adrenal insufficiency [19]. Hypothetically, obesity may result from insufficient hypothalamic melanocyte-stimulating hormone, which may regulate appetite when bound to the melanocortin-4 receptor (MC4R).

Melanocortin-4 receptor gene mutations also cause an autosomal-recessive form of obesity in mice and are found in some morbidly obese humans [20,21]. MC4R deficiency represents the most commonly known monogenic disorder causing morbid obesity [22]. Heterozygotes for this mutation may or may not express obesity. MC4R-mutant subjects have a parallel increase in lean body mass and height and less hyperphagia than subjects with leptin deficiency do, and they demonstrate early-onset hyperinsulinemia [14].

An autosomal-dominant form of mouse obesity, the yellow mouse, results from a mutation in the agouti gene that causes over-expression of the agouti protein, inhibits normal expression of the hypothalamic melanocortin-4 receptor, and results in uninhibited appetite [23]. This mechanism has not yet been extensively described in humans.

There is also an ongoing search for more peripheral genetic causes of obesity. Genes that control the number of adipocytes, how they store fat, and how lean body cells expend energy are being studied. A family of uncoupling proteins (UCPs) has been described that allows cells to waste energy as heat rather than store or use energy [18]. There is a strong genetic component to the amount of weight gained during experimental overfeeding, which is not explained by resting energy expenditure. This event has been attributed to "nonexercise activity thermogenesis," which results in calories being burned by such mechanisms as increased fidgeting, maintenance of posture, and other activities of daily living [24]. In other words, some humans expend more energy just living and thus are resistant to weight gain.

The economic and sociologic impacts of obesity are rising in conjunction with the incidence. Obesity is considered today to be the second most important public health problem in the United States, surpassed only by tobacco use. In 2000, tobacco use was estimated to be responsible annually for 435,000 deaths and obesity for 400,000 deaths [25]. Although obesity is more common in African-American than in white men and women in the United States, early mortality is more commonly associated with obesity in whites [26].

Five obesity-related diseases account for the health care cost burden of the epidemic, estimated at $99 billion in 1995 [27]. Diseases include hypertension, hyperlipidemia, type 2 diabetes, coronary artery disease, and stroke. Obesity is a major contributor to the insulin resistant syndrome (IRS), also known as the metabolic syndrome or dysmetabolic syndrome. The third report of the National Cholesterol Education Program Expert Panel on Detection, Evaluation, and Treatment of High Blood Cholesterol in Adults [28] defines IRS as the presence of three or more of the following:

1. Abdominal obesity: waist circumference of more than 102 cm in men and more than 88 cm in women
2. Hypertriglyceridemia ($\geq$150 mg/dL)
3. Low level of high-density lipoprotein cholesterol ($\leq$40 mg/dL in men and $\leq$50 mg/dL in women)
4. High blood pressure ($\geq$135/85 mm Hg)
5. High level of fasting glucose ($\geq$110 mg/dL)

Childhood BMI is the most significant predictor of IRS in young adulthood [29]. Offspring of diabetic parents, regardless of race, displayed excess body fat and an accelerated progression of IRS characteristics from childhood to young adulthood.

There are significant racial differences in the relationship between obesity and diseases. African-Americans have a less athrogenic lipid pattern than do whites but higher rates of coronary heart disease and stroke. The prevalence of hypertension is greatest in African-Americans, and the prevalence of type II diabetes is greatest in Mexican Americans [8]. At any given age, mortality at the highest BMI is greatest in whites [25].

A 1-year study [30] of health care costs for obese adults enrolled in an HMO reported nearly twice the cost of prescription drugs and almost four times the hospitalization rate compared with nonobese members. The median number of outpatient visits was also higher, with greater individual variability among the obese. The prescription drugs most used by the obese included antihypertensive agents, calcium channel blockers, β blockers, diuretics, intranasal allergic rhinitis preparations, asthma medications, ulcer medications, thyroid drugs, and narcotic and non-narcotic pain medications. It has been shown that yearly expenditures and total individual Medicare expenditures increase with increasing BMI in middle age, further emphasizing the economic implications of this epidemic [31].

Highly associated with obesity, diabetes itself has been linked with myriad associated disorders including retinopathy, neuropathy, microvascular disease, large vessel disease, and cardiac disorders. Obesity is associated with postmenopausal breast cancer and cancers of the endometrium, colon, pancreas, esophagus, kidney, gallbladder, and gastric cardia [32]. Insulin resistance and hyperinsulinemia have been postulated to be the reason, as may be altered sex hormone levels [33].

With no end in sight to the obesity epidemic, the American Medical Association has taken upon itself the task of publicizing this condition strongly. A major report is due from the AMA Council on Scientific Affairs in June, 2005. The AMA Web site is replete with practice directions, statistics, and links to other important sites. Dietary and physical activity recommendations are widely available. The news media are tuned into the problem, and information is freely available to the public. The McDonald's Company has been sued, and the Arby's Company has been publicly chastised. It will be interesting to see whether recent trends can be reversed with all this media attention.

References

[1] National Institutes of Health. Clinical guidelines on the identification, evaluation and treatment of overweight and obesity in adults: the evidence report. Obes Res 1998;6(Suppl 2):51S–209S.

[2] World Health Organization. Turning the tide of malnutrition: responding to the challenge of the 21st century. Available at: www.who.int/nut/documents/nhd_brochure.pdf. Accessed December 3, 2004.

[3] Mokdad AH, Ford ES, Bowman BA, et al. Prevalence of obesity, diabetes and obesity-related health risk factors. JAMA 2003;289:76–9.

[4] Flegal KM, Carroll MD, Ogden CL, et al. Prevalence and trends in obesity among US adults 1999–2000. JAMA 2002;288:1723–7.

[5] Freedman DS, Khan LK, Serdula MK, et al. Trends and correlates of class 3 obesity in the United States from 1990–2000. JAMA 2002;288:1758–61.

[6] National Center for Chronic Disease Prevention and Health Promotion. Obesity trends among US adults between 1985 and 2003. Available at: www.cdc.gov/nccdphp/dnpa/obesity/. Accessed December 2, 2004.

[7] Cooney KA, Gruber SB. Hyperglycemia, obesity and cancer risks on the horizon. JAMA 2005; 293:235–6.

[8] Crossrow N, Falkner B. Race/ethnic issues in obesity and obesity-related comorbidities. J Clin Endocrinol Metab 2004;89:2590–4.

[9] Goel MS, McCarthy EP, Phillips RS, et al. Obesity among US immigrant subgroups by duration of residence. JAMA 2004;292:2860–7.

[10] Childhood obesity in the United States: facts and figures. Fact sheet, September 2004. Institute of Medicine Web site. Available at: www.iom.edu. Accessed March 28, 2005.

[11] Schwimmer JB, Burwinkle TM, Varni JW. Health related quality of life of severely obese children and adolescents. JAMA 2003;289:1813–9.

[12] Stunkard AJ, Harris JR, Pederson NL, et al. The body-mass index of twins who have been reared apart. N Engl J Med 1990;322:1483–7.

[13] Allison DB, Kaprio J, Korkeila M, et al. The heritability of body mass index among an international sample of monozygotic twins reared apart. Int J Obes Relat Metab Disord 1996; 20:501–6.

[14] O'Rahilly S, Farooqi IS, Yeo GSH, et al. Minireview: human obesity–lessons from monogenetic disorders. Endocrinology 2003;144:3757–64.

[15] Physical activity trends: United States 1990–1998. MMWR Morb Mortal Wkly Rep 2001;50: 166–9.

[16] Perusse L, Chagnon YC, Weisnagel J, et al. The human obesity gene map: the 1998 update. Obes Res 1999;7:111–29.

[17] Farooqi HS, Matarese G, Lord GM, et al. Beneficial effects of leptin on obesity, T cell hypo-responsiveness and neuroendocrine/metabolic dysfunction of human congenital leptin deficiency. J Clin Invest 2002;110:1093–103.

[18] Yanovski JA, Yanovski SZ. Recent advances in obesity research. JAMA 1999;282:1504–6.

[19] Krude H, Biebermann H, Luck W, et al. Severe early-onset obesity, adrenal insufficiency and red hair pigmentation caused by POMC mutations in humans. Nat Genet 1998;19:155–7.

[20] Vaisse C, Clement K, Guy-Grand B, et al. A frameshift mutation in human MC4R is associated with a dominant form of obesity. Nat Genet 1998;20:113–4.

[21] Yeo GS, Farooki IS, Aminian S, et al. A frameshift mutation in human MC4R is associated with a dominantly inherited human obesity. Nat Genet 1998;20:111–2.

[22] Mergen M, Mergen H, Ozata M, et al. A novel melanocortin 4 receptor (MC4R) gene mutation associated with morbid obesity. J Clin Endocrinol Metab 2001;86:3448.

[23] Lu D, Willard D, Patel IR, et al. Agouti protein is an antagonist of the melanocytic-stimulating-hormone receptor. Nature 1994;371:799–802.

[24] Levine JA, Eberhardt NL, Jensen MD. Role of nonexercise activity thermogenesis in resistance to fat gain in humans. Science 1999;283:212–4.

[25] Calle EE, Thun MJ, Petrelli JM, et al. Body mass index and mortality in a prospective cohort of US adults. N Engl J Med 1999;341:1097–105.

[26] Mokdad AH, Marks JS, Stroup DF, et al. Actual causes of death in the United States, 2000. JAMA 2004;291:1238–45.

[27] Wolf AM, Colditz GA. Current estimates of the economic cost of obesity in the United States. Obes Res 1998;6:97–106.

[28] National Institutes of Health. Third report of the national cholesterol education program expert panel on detection, evaluation and treatment of high blood cholesterol in adults (adult treatment panel III). Bethesda, MD: National Institutes of Health; 2001 [NIH publication 01–3670].

[29] Srinivasan SR, Meyers L, Berensen GS for the Bogalusa Heart Study. Predictability of childhood adiposity and insulin for developing insulin resistance syndrome (Syndrome X) in young adulthood. Diabetes 2000;51:204–9.

[30] Raebel MA, Malone DC, Conner DA, et al. Health services use and health care costs of obese and nonobese individuals. Arch Intern Med 2004;164:2135–40.

[31] Daviglus MI, Liu K, Yan LL, et al. Relation of body mass index in young adulthood and middle age to Medicare expenditures in older age. JAMA 2004;292:2743–9.

[32] Calle EE, Kaaks R. Overweight, obesity and cancer: epidemiological evidence and proposed mechanisms. Nat Rev Cancer 2004;94:579–91.

[33] Cooney KA, Gruber SB. Hyperglycemia, obesity and cancer risks on the horizon. JAMA 2005; 293:235–6.

ELSEVIER
SAUNDERS

Anesthesiology Clin N Am
23 (2005) 405–420

ANESTHESIOLOGY
CLINICS OF
NORTH AMERICA

Demographics and Diagnosis of Obstructive Sleep Apnea

Tracey Stierer, MD[a],*, Naresh M. Punjabi, MD, PhD[b]

[a]*Department of Anesthesiology and Critical Care Medicine,*
Johns Hopkins University School of Medicine, 601 North Caroline Street, B165A,
Baltimore, Maryland 21287-0712, USA
[b]*Department of Medicine, Johns Hopkins University School of Medicine, 601 North Caroline Street,*
B165A, Baltimore, Maryland 21287-0712, USA

Obstructive sleep apnea (OSA) is a common disorder characterized by recurrent episodes of a complete or partial collapse of the upper airway during sleep. The cessation or reduction in respiratory airflow may be associated with a decrease in oxygen saturation or arousal from sleep. Patients with OSA present with a constellation of nocturnal symptoms that may include loud disruptive snoring, breathing pauses (apneas), choking, gasping, and frequent awakenings. Daytime symptoms may include excessive daytime sleepiness, fatigue, irritability, and deficits in attention and memory. Data from the Wisconsin Sleep Cohort Study [1] show that sleep apnea affects 2% to 4% of middle-aged working adults in the general population. Despite the increasing body of literature in which the adverse health consequences and public health impact of sleep apnea are recognized, a considerable number of affected individuals still remain undiagnosed [2,3]. It is now well accepted that the adverse health consequences from OSA are attributable to two fundamental abnormalities that occur during sleep. First, the cessation or reduction in respiratory airflow leads to abnormalities in gas exchange, resulting in hypoxemia and hypercapnia. Second, the repetitive arousals caused by obstructive apneas and hypopneas result in sleep fragmentation and the loss of restorative sleep. The increase in cardiovascular and noncardiovascular morbidity appears to be mediated by the complex inter-

---

* Corresponding author.
E-mail address: tstiere@jhmi.edu (T. Stierer).

0889-8537/05/$ – see front matter © 2005 Elsevier Inc. All rights reserved.
doi:10.1016/j.atc.2005.03.009   *anesthesiology.theclinics.com*

action between abnormalities of gas exchange, fragmentation of sleep, and the mechanical effects of repetitive upper airway closure.

Compared with patients without OSA, those with the disease may be at a higher risk for adverse perioperative outcomes, including death [4,5]. Frequently associated with difficult mask ventilation and intubation, the surgical patient with a formal diagnosis of OSA presents a major challenge to the anesthesiologist [6,7]. Life-threatening problems can arise with respect to tracheal intubation and extubation and the provision of satisfactory postoperative analgesia. Attempts to ventilate a patient using a mask after the induction of anesthesia may be unsuccessful and lead to the need for an emergency airway or death. An additional challenge is the perioperative management of individuals who may have moderate to severe OSA but remain undiagnosed. Therefore, knowledge of factors associated with an increased risk of OSA is vital to the perioperative assessment and anesthetic plan. This article reviews the terminology of OSA and the associated diagnostic tests and provides an overview of the risk factors for this chronic condition.

Disease definition and diagnosis

A sleep study or a polysomnogram is the standard diagnostic test for OSA. The test involves simultaneous recordings of multiple physiologic signals, including the right and left electro-oculograms, the submental electromyogram, and the electroencephalogram. Collectively, these surface recordings are used to distinguish wakefulness from sleep and determine the distribution of different sleep stages over the course of the night. Additionally, breathing patterns are assessed with measurements of respiratory effort (assessed with impedance plethysmography), airflow, and oxygen saturation. Changes in airflow are recorded with either an oronasal thermistor (a probe sensitive to temperature changes that occur with breathing) or a nasal cannula configured to monitor pressure changes in the nasal airway. Other measures include the assessment of body position and continuous monitoring of the electrocardiogram to detect occurrence of cardiac arrhythmias during sleep. The analysis of the polysomnogram for OSA requires identifying abnormal or disordered breathing patterns during sleep.

There are two basic types of disordered breathing events: apneas and hypopneas. An apnea is defined as the complete cessation of airflow for at least 10 seconds. A hypopnea is defined as a reduction in airflow associated with an electroencephalogram arousal or a decrease in oxygen saturation [8]. Commonly used definitions of hypopnea are based on an airflow reduction of 25% or 50% and an oxygen saturation reduction of 3% or 4% (Table 1). Disordered breathing events are further classified into obstructive, central, or mixed events. The classification of an abnormal breathing event depends on whether there is evidence of respiratory effort in the absence of airflow. An obstructive event is defined as the absence of airflow despite continued effort. In contrast, a central event is defined as the absence of airflow without associated effort. A mixed

Table 1
Terminology of obstructive sleep apnea

Term	Definition
Disordered breathing event	
Apnea	Complete cessation of airflow for at least ten seconds
Hypopnea	Reduction in airflow associated with electroencephalographic arousal or oxygen desaturation. Common definitions of reduction in airflow include: 50% decrease from baseline, 25% decrease from baseline, or any discernable reduction in airflow from baseline. Common thresholds used to defined oxygen desaturation include a 3% or 4% drop from baseline values.
Type of disordered breathing event	
Obstructive	An event with absence of airflow but with continued respiratory effort
Central	An event with absence of airflow and no respiratory effort
Mixed	An event with characteristics of an obstructive and mixed event. These events typically start with a period that meets the criteria for a central event but will end with respiratory effort without airflow
Indices on disordered breathing severity	
Apnea-hypopnea Index	Number of apneas and hypopneas per hour of total sleep time
Apnea index	Number of apneas per hour of total sleep time
Hypopnea index	Number of hypopneas per hour of total sleep time
Central apnea index	Number of central apneas per hour of total sleep time

event manifests characteristics of an obstructive and a central event. Mixed events typically start with a period that meets the criteria for a central event but end with increasing effort but without associated airflow. Traces illustrating normal and abnormal (obstructive, mixed, and central) breathing patterns during sleep are shown in Figs. 1–4.

A number of indices of disease severity are derived from the polysomnogram (see Table 1). The apnea-hypopnea index (AHI), which is the number of apneas and hypopneas that occur per hour of sleep, is commonly used to quantify OSA severity. Other measures that are commonly reported are an apnea index (number of apneas per hour), a hypopnea index (number of hypopneas per hour), and an arousal index (number of arousals per hour of sleep). Some laboratories also provide more detailed information, including a breakdown of these indices for nonrapid and rapid eye movement (NREM) sleep, and whether there are differences with body position (side versus back). These subdivisions are clinically useful because they provide insight into the clinical variants of OSA (eg, positional apnea and REM-related apnea). Finally, measures of oxyhemoglobin saturation and the degree of nocturnal desaturation are also included. Presently, there is no consensus as to what threshold in the disease-defining metric should be used to distinguish the "normal" from the "diseased" state (ie, apnea-hypopnea index and apnea index). An AHI of 5 events or more per hour is commonly used as the disease-defining threshold in most clinical and research settings. However, ongoing epidemiologic studies have shown that even lower

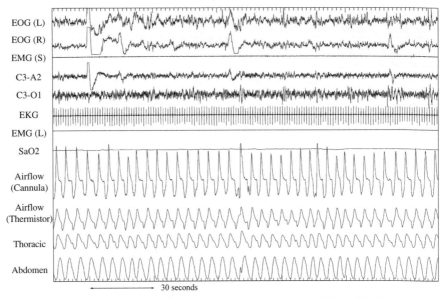

Channels recorded: Electrooculogram (EOG) from both eyes; Electromyogram (EMG) of chin (S) and leg (Ł), electroencephalogram (EEG) from standard locations C3-A2, C3-O1; electrocardiogram (ECG); oxygen saturation (SaO2); airflow (cannula and thermistor); respiratory effort (thoracic and abdomen)

Fig. 1. Polysomnographic tracings of normal breathing during sleep. Channels recorded were electrooculogram (EOG) from both eyes; electromyogram (EMG) of chin (S) and leg (L); electroencephalogram (EEG) from standard locations C3-A2 and C3-O1; electrocardiogram (ECG); oxygen saturation (SaO2); airflow (Cannula and Thermistor); and respiratory (Thoracic and Abdomen).

levels of disordered breathing are associated with an increased risk of cardiovascular disease [9,10].

Population prevalence of obstructive sleep apnea

Estimates of OSA prevalence in the general population vary widely depending on the population studied, the methods used to measure sleep, and the definition of disordered breathing. Earlier studies [11,12] have used an apnea index of greater than five or 10 events per hour to define OSA. As the clinical impact of hypopneas was recognized, the combined AHI index became the standard metric for diagnosing OSA. However, the issue of a specific AHI threshold to define the disease state remains unresolved. Obviously, estimates of OSA prevalence will vary significantly, depending on the AHI threshold that discriminates normal from abnormal. Inconsistencies across studies in the methods used for monitoring sleep and breathing also contribute to variability in the available estimates of the prevalence of OSA. Two common approaches used to document disordered breathing during sleep are oximetry and full-night polysomnography. Population-based studies that have used oximetry to assess respiratory abnor-

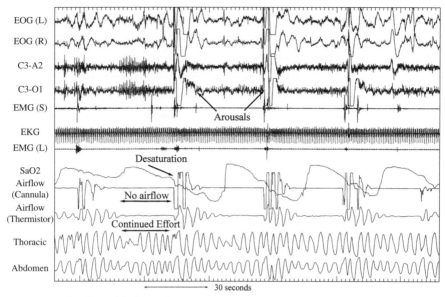

Channels recorded: Electrooculogram (EOG) from both eyes; Electromyogram (EMG) of chin (S) and leg (L), electroencephalogram (EEG) from standard locations C3-A2, C3-O1; electrocardiogram (ECG); oxygen saturation (SaO2); airflow (cannula and thermistor); respiratory effort (thoracic and abdomen)

Fig. 2. Polysomnographic tracings of obstructive sleep apnea. Channels recorded were electrooculogram (EOG) from both eyes; electromyogram (EMG) of chin (S) and leg (L); electroencephalogram (EEG) from standard locations C3-A2 and C3-O1; electrocardiogram (ECG); oxygen saturation (SaO2); airflow (Cannula and Thermistor); and respiratory (Thoracic and Abdomen).

malities show that the prevalence of OSA is generally lower than those studies that have used polysomnography because disordered breathing events without oxygen desaturation are not identified with the former approach. Finally, differences in study design and sample population are other sources of variability in the reported prevalence of OSA. Therefore, estimates of OSA prevalence should be interpreted with careful attention to the above methodological issues.

Of the studies available on the population prevalence of OSA, three studies have used a laboratory polysomnogram to identify the presence of apneas and hypopneas during sleep. These studies have generally provided convergent findings. Data from the Wisconsin Sleep Cohort Study [1] suggest that approximately 4% of women and 9% of men in the United States (ages 40 to 65 years) have moderate OSA, defined as an AHI of 15 or more events per hour during sleep. Similar estimates of OSA prevalence have also been reported by Bixler et al [13,14] in a sample of 1741 individuals recruited from the general population. These authors noted that 2% of women and 4% of men in their sample had moderate to severe sleep apnea (AHI $\geq$15 events/h). Confirming evidence for the relatively high prevalence of sleep apnea also comes from studies conducted outside the United States. In a sample of 30- to 70-year-old subjects, Duran et al [15] noted a 7% and 14% prevalence of sleep apnea in men and

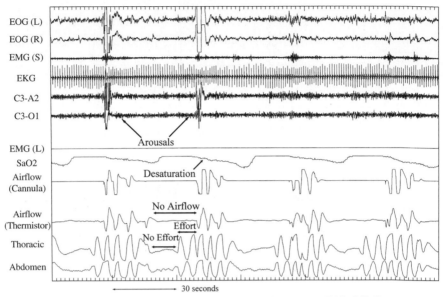

Channels recorded: Electrooculogram (EOG) from both eyes; Electromyogram (EMG) of chin (S)
and leg (L), electroencephalogram (EEG) from standard locations C3-A2, C3-O1; electrocardiogram (ECG);
oxygen saturation (SaO2); airflow (cannula and thermistor); respiratory effort (thoracic and abdomen)

Fig. 3. Polysomnographic tracings of central sleep apnea. Channels recorded were electro-oculogram
(EOG) from both eyes; electromyogram (EMG) of chin (S) and leg (L); electroencephalogram (EEG)
from standard locations C3-A2 and C3-O1; electrocardiogram (ECG); oxygen saturation (SaO2);
airflow (Cannula and Thermistor); and respiratory (Thoracic and Abdomen).

women, respectively, based on a sample of subjects recruited from Spain. Obviously, prevalence estimates change as the demographics of the population
studied are altered. Most, if not all, cross-sectional surveys of clinic [16–24]
and population-based samples [25–31] show that obesity is the strongest risk
factor for OSA. Other factors that increase the risk for sleep apnea include male
gender [1,14,32,33], increasing age [13,15,33,34], race [34–36], and family
history [37–44]. The following sections describe factors that are known to increase the risk for OSA and can be used in the case identification of undiagnosed individuals.

Risk factors for obstructive sleep apnea

The occurrence of pharyngeal collapse during sleep, the fundamental basis
for OSA, suggests that sleep onset is associated with functional alterations in
the upper airway that reduce its patency and increase resistance to airflow. Although the precise mechanisms of upper-airway collapse during sleep are not
well defined, two fundamental features of the pathogenesis of upper-airway obstruction are clear. First, patients with OSA manifest structural abnormalities of

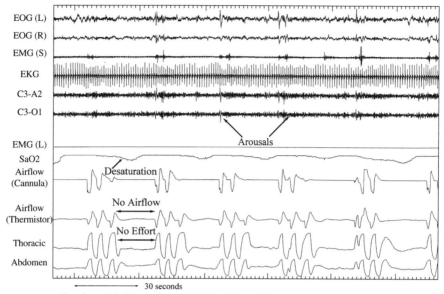

Channels recorded: Electrooculogram (EOG) from both eyes; Electromyogram (EMG) of chin (S)
and leg (L), electroencephalogram (EEG) from standard locations C3-A2, C3-O1; electrocardiogram (ECG);
oxygen saturation (SaO2); airflow (cannula and thermistor); respiratory effort (thoracic and abdomen)

Fig. 4. Polysomnographic tracings of mixed sleep apnea. Channels recorded were electro-oculogram
(EOG) from both eyes; electromyogram (EMG) of chin (S) and leg (L); electroencephalogram (EEG)
from standard locations C3-A2 and C3-O1; electrocardiogram (ECG); oxygen saturation (SaO2);
airflow (Cannula and Thermistor); and respiratory (Thoracic and Abdomen).

the upper airway. An increased volume of retropalatal soft tissue, particularly in
the lateral dimension, contributes to airway narrowing [45,46]. Second, patients
also appear to have a defect in upper-airway neuromuscular activation [47–51].
Whether structural abnormalities or alterations in upper-airway neural control
constitute the primary abnormality remains to be determined. Several factors have
been shown to increase the risk for OSA, including obesity, male gender, age,
race, family history, craniofacial abnormalities, and the use of alcohol or other
pharmacologic agents.

Obesity

    Evidence for the increased risk for OSA in overweight and obese individu-
als comes from numerous clinic and population-based studies that demonstrate
either a high prevalence of obesity in patients with OSA or a high prevalence of
OSA in overweight and obese individuals [16–31]. Polysomnographic evaluation of morbidly obese subjects without sleep-related complaints shows that at
least 40% of men and 3% of women have OSA that is severe enough to warrant
treatment [52]. Data from the Wisconsin Sleep Cohort Study [1] indicate that an
increase of one standard deviation in the body mass index (BMI) is associated

with an increased risk of OSA of almost fourfold. Results of the ongoing multi-center Sleep Heart Health Study [33] also confirm that obesity is an important risk factor for OSA and that the effects of excess body weight are modified by age and gender. Finally, studies of weight loss have also shown that obesity plays a causal role in the pathogenesis of OSA. Significant improvements in the AHI, nocturnal desaturation, and sleep architecture have been documented with dietary [53–58] and surgical weight loss [59–62].

The mechanisms by which obesity increases the risk of OSA are not well known. Excess body mass is associated with alterations in upper-airway structure [17,18]. Increases in neck circumference and fat deposition around the upper airway in overweight and obese subjects can decrease upper airway size [45]. Collapsibility of the upper airway occurs more frequently in obese than nonobese subjects [56]. Obesity, particularly central obesity, is associated with reductions in lung volume [63] that can alter upper-airway collapsibility [64–68] and predispose an individual to OSA. Thus, by imposing mechanical loads on the upper airway and the respiratory system, excess body weight can alter upper-airway structure and function and thereby increase the propensity for airflow obstruction during sleep.

Gender

It is well established that male gender is a major risk factor for OSA. Early clinical observations have shown that men have an almost 10-fold greater risk for OSA compared with women [69,70]. Recent epidemiologic studies [32,33], however, have failed to substantiate the strong male predisposition and indicate a 2- to 3-fold greater risk for OSA in men compared with women. The physiologic basis for the increased risk of OSA in men is poorly understood. Differences in upper-airway structure and function have been hypothesized to account for the disparity in OSA prevalence between men and women. Although previous studies [71–73] addressing the affects of gender on upper-airway cross-sectional area and size reported inconsistent results, accumulating data indicate that the minimum cross-sectional area of the upper airway may be similar in both genders [74,75]. Thus, anatomical differences alone may not completely account for the male predisposition to OSA. Physiologic data [76] suggest that the upper airway in women may be less collapsible than in men, a finding that has been attributed to female sex hormones [77,78]. However, the data regarding the effect of sex hormones on OSA are minimal, and there are significant gaps in our understanding of the role of these hormones in the pathogenesis of pharyngeal collapse during sleep. Nevertheless, male gender is an important risk factor for OSA.

Age

Several cross-sectional surveys from community samples indicate that the prevalence of OSA increases steadily with advancing age. In one of the earliest studies, Ancoli-Israel et al [79] examined a random sample of 427 65- to 99-year-old men and women using inductive plethysmography and actigraphy (the measurement of body motion) during sleep. Using an AHI of 10 or more events per hour as the criterion for diagnosis, 70% of men and 62% of women were found to have OSA. Subsequent studies from several large population-based cohorts have confirmed the high prevalence of OSA in older adults. In a probability sample from two Pennsylvania counties, Bixler et al [13,14] noted that the risk for OSA in older adults was two to three times higher than in middle-aged adults. The prevalence of OSA (defined as an AHI $\geq$15 events/h) for men in the 65- to 100-year-old group was 23.9%, whereas the prevalence in the 45- to 64-year-old group was 11.8% [13]. In women, the prevalence of OSA (defined as an AHI $\geq$15 events/h) in the 45- to 64-year-old group was 2.0%, whereas in the 65- to 100-year-old group, the prevalence was 7.0% [14]. The association between the risk of OSA and increasing age was confirmed by Duran et al [15] in a population cohort from Spain. In a group of 400 individuals characterized with an in-laboratory polysomnogram, the authors found that the OSA prevalence was lowest in the 30- to 39-year-old age group (7.6% in men and 1.7% in women) and dramatically increased in the 60-to 70-year-old group (32.2% in men and 25.6% in women). Currently, the mechanisms underlying the association between advancing age and OSA are poorly understood. Possible explanations include age-related changes in upper-airway caliber [80–83], attenuation in the ventilatory response to hypoxia and hypercapnia [84–87], decreases in functional activity of the upper airway [88], and an increase in the variability of ventilation during sleep [81].

Race

The prevalence and severity of OSA also have been found to be associated with race. Data from the Cleveland family study [35] indicate that African-Americans are at an increased risk for OSA compared with whites, independent of gender and body weight (odds ratio, 1.88; 95% confidence interval [CI]:1.03–3.52). Although the risk for OSA was also noted to be higher with increasing age for African-Americans than whites [34], recent data from the multicenter Sleep Heart Health Study [1] failed to confirm the increased propensity for OSA in African-Americans after accounting for various confounding factors, including age, gender, and body weight [33]. The reasons for variable estimates of OSA risk in African-Americans across different studies are not entirely clear. Nevertheless, it appears that other ethnic groups may have a higher predisposition to OSA. Epidemiologic investigations by Ip et al [89,90] reveal that the prevalence of OSA in Chinese men and women is 4.1% and 2.1%, respectively. Although these estimates of OSA prevalence are similar to those noted in the Wisconsin sleep cohort study, the clinically significant differences in the distribution of BMI between Asians and whites suggest that other factors such as differences in craniofacial structure may play a significant role in the pathogenesis of OSA across different racial groups [91].

Craniofacial abnormalities

Cephalometric analyses reveal a number of skeletal and soft tissue abnormalities in patients with OSA compared with age- and gender-matched controls [91–99]. Although a detailed discussion of the role of craniofacial structure in the pathophysiology of OSA is outside the scope of this review, features such as retrognathia, enlarged tongue or soft palate, inferiorly positioned hyoid bone, maxillary and mandibular retroposition, and decreased posterior airway space are commonly found in patients with OSA. The relative contribution of craniofacial abnormalities to the pathogenesis of upper-airway collapse during sleep may be different in lean and obese patients [97–99]. Abnormalities of bony structures may have a larger influence on upper-airway mechanics in nonobese patients, whereas abnormalities in soft-tissue structures may contribute minimally in obese patients. Abnormal craniofacial and soft tissue structures have been shown to increase upper-airway collapsibility during sleep and thus may increase the risk for OSA [100].

Family history

Several studies [38,39,101] have suggested that family history also may influence the risk of OSA. Familial clustering was initially demonstrated in several families with multiple affected members and by the high prevalence of OSA symptoms in first-degree relatives of affected individuals [40]. Subsequent studies using either abbreviated methods for monitoring respiration during sleep [42,44] or full montage polysomnography [41,43] have confirmed the familial aggregation of OSA [43,44]. The increased risk in family members appears to be independent of other inherited factors such as obesity. Recent work using whole genome scans in the Cleveland Family Study [102,103] has shown that there may in fact be specific chromosomal linkages that may increase the susceptibility to OSA. A familial tendency toward OSA could be attributable to inheritable factors such as craniofacial features or respiratory neural control mechanisms that decrease upper-airway collapsibility during sleep. However, presently, the specific determinants that increase the OSA risk in families are not known.

Alcohol consumption

Alcohol consumption has been associated with an increased risk of OSA. Alcohol ingestion can induce apneic activity in previously normal or asymptomatic individuals [104–106]. In patients with OSA, alcohol intake can prolong apneic duration and worsen the severity of associated hypoxemia [107–110]. The mechanisms by which alcohol induces or worsens pharyngeal collapse have not been fully characterized. Experimental studies in both animals and humans indicate that alcohol reduces respiratory motor output to the upper airway, resulting in oropharyngeal hypotonia [106,111–113]. Although the data on patient factors that promote upper-airway collapse with alcohol are limited, the effect of alcohol appears to be more pronounced in men than in women [112].

Summary

OSA is a prevalent and often undiagnosed condition in the general population. There are several underlying reasons for the disparity between the prevalence of OSA and the current level of clinical recognition. The standard diagnostic test (polysomnogram) is labor intensive, time consuming, and available primarily through centers that specialize in sleep medicine. This limitation in the diagnostic infrastructure coupled with the fact that most physicians fail to recognize sleep-related symptoms has limited the number of individuals that have been appropriately identified. The lack of recognition of patients with undiagnosed OSA presents a dilemma for the anesthesia care provider. When the diagnosis of OSA is known, traditional provisions for management have included a specific plan and the equipment to secure the difficult airway and the ability to monitor the patient postoperatively, with increased surveillance for obstructive apneic episodes. These additional resources can be arranged, and the surgical procedure can be scheduled in an appropriate location of care to ensure the safety of the patient . Although screening for OSA is commonly performed in the preoperative setting, standardized methods for identifying affected but undiagnosed individuals are lacking. The availability of a simple and valid screening method that identifies individuals with undiagnosed OSA is of paramount significance to streamline the perioperative management of such patients and deter adverse postoperative sequelae.

References

[1] Young T, Palta M, Dempsey J, et al. The occurrence of sleep-disordered breathing among middle-aged adults. N Engl J Med 1993;328:1230–5.

[2] Young T, Evans L, Finn L, et al. Estimation of the clinically diagnosed proportion of sleep apnea syndrome in middle-aged men and women. Sleep 1997;20:705–6.

[3] Kapur V, Strohl KP, Redline S, et al. Underdiagnosis of sleep apnea syndrome in US communities. Sleep Breath 2002;6:49–54.

[4] Ostermeier AM, Roizen MF, Hautkappe M, et al. Three sudden postoperative respiratory arrests associated with epidural opioids in patients with sleep apnea. Anesth Analg 1997;85: 452–60.

[5] Gupta RM, Parvizi J, Hanssen AD, et al. Postoperative complications in patients with obstructive sleep apnea syndrome undergoing hip or knee replacement: a case-control study. Mayo Clin Proc 2001;76:897–905.

[6] Hiremath AS, Hillman DR, James AL, et al. Relationship between difficult tracheal intubation and obstructive sleep apnoea. Br J Anaesth 1998;80:606–11.

[7] Benumof JL. Obstructive sleep apnea in the adult obese patient: implications for airway management. Anesthesiol Clin North America 2002;20:789–811.

[8] American Academy of Sleep Medicine Task Force. Sleep-related breathing disorders in adults:

recommendations for syndrome definition and measurement techniques in clinical research. Sleep Med 1999;22:667–89.

[9] Nieto FJ, Young TB, Lind BK, et al for the Sleep Heart Health Study. Association of sleep-disordered breathing, sleep apnea, and hypertension in a large community-based study. JAMA 2000;283:1829–36.

[10] Shahar E, Whitney CW, Redline S, et al. Sleep-disordered breathing and cardiovascular disease: cross-sectional results of the Sleep Heart Health Study. Am J Respir Crit Care Med 2001;163: 19–25.

[11] Lavie P. Incidence of sleep apnea in a presumably healthy working population: a significant relationship with excessive daytime sleepiness. Sleep 1983;6:312–8.

[12] Peter JH, Siegrist J, Podszus T, et al. Prevalence of sleep apnea in healthy industrial workers. Wein Klin Wochenschr 1985;63:807–11.

[13] Bixler EO, Vgontzas AN, Ten Have T, et al. Effects of age on sleep apnea in men: I. prevalence and severity. Am J Respir Crit Care Med 1998;157:144–8.

[14] Bixler EO, Vgontzas AN, Lin HM, et al. Prevalence of sleep-disordered breathing in women: effects of gender. Am J Respir Crit Care Med 2001;163:608–13.

[15] Duran J, Esnaola S, Rubio R, et al. Obstructive sleep apnea-hypopnea and related clinical features in a population-based sample of subjects aged 30 to 70 yr. Am J Respir Crit Care Med 2001;163:685–9.

[16] Davies RJ, Stradling JR. The relationship between neck circumference, radiographic pharyngeal anatomy, and the obstructive sleep apnoea syndrome. Eur Respir J 1990;3:509–14.

[17] Katz I, Stradling J, Slutsky AS, et al. Do patients with obstructive sleep apnea have thick necks? Am Rev Respir Dis 1990;141:1228–31.

[18] Davies RJ, Ali NJ, Stradling JR. Neck circumference and other clinical features in the diagnosis of the obstructive sleep apnoea syndrome. Thorax 1992;47:101–5.

[19] Hoffstein V, Mateika S. Differences in abdominal and neck circumferences in patients with and without obstructive sleep apnoea. Eur Respir J 1992;5:377–81.

[20] Grunstein R, Wilcox I, Yang TS, et al. Snoring and sleep apnoea in men: association with central obesity and hypertension. Int J Obes Relat Metab Disord 1993;17:533–40.

[21] Levinson PD, McGarvey ST, Carlisle CC, et al. Adiposity and cardiovascular risk factors in men with obstructive sleep apnea. Chest 1993;103:1336–42.

[22] Richman RM, Elliott LM, Burns CM, et al. The prevalence of obstructive sleep apnoea in an obese female population. Int J Obes Relat Metab Disord 1994;18:173–7.

[23] Millman RP, Carlisle CC, McGarvey ST, et al. Body fat distribution and sleep apnea severity in women. Chest 1995;7:362–6.

[24] Shinohara E, Kihara S, Yamashita S, et al. Visceral fat accumulation as an important risk factor for obstructive sleep apnoea syndrome in obese subjects. J Intern Med 1997;241:11–8.

[25] Stradling JR, Crosby JH. Predictors and prevalence of obstructive sleep apnoea and snoring in 1001 middle aged men. Thorax 1991;46:85–90.

[26] Bearpark H, Elliott L, Grunstein R, et al. Occurrence and correlates of sleep disordered breathing in the Australian town of Busselton: a preliminary analysis. Sleep 1993;16(Suppl 8):S3–5.

[27] Jennum P, Sjol A. Snoring, sleep apnoea and cardiovascular risk factors: the MONICA II study. Int J Epidemiol 1993;22:439–44.

[28] Ferini-Strambi L, Zucconi M, Palazzi S, et al. Snoring and nocturnal oxygen desaturations in an Italian middle-aged male population: epidemiologic study with an ambulatory device. Chest 1994;105:1759–64.

[29] Olson LG, King MT, Hensley MJ, et al. A community study of snoring and sleep-disordered breathing: prevalence. Am J Respir Crit Care Med 1995;152:711–6.

[30] Ferini-Strambi L, Zucconi M, Castronovo V, et al. Snoring and sleep apnea: a population study in Italian women. Sleep 1999;22:859–64.

[31] Newman AB, Nieto FJ, Guidry U, et al. Relation of sleep-disordered breathing to cardiovascular disease risk factors: the Sleep Heart Health Study. Am J Epidemiol 2001;154:50–9.

[32] Redline S, Kump K, Tishler PV, et al. Gender differences in sleep disordered breathing in a community-based sample. Am J Respir Crit Care Med 1994;149:722–6.

[33] Young T, Shahar E, Nieto FJ, et al. Predictors of sleep-disordered breathing in community-dwelling adults: the Sleep Heart Health Study. Arch Intern Med 2002;162:893–900.

[34] Ancoli-Israel S, Klauber MR, Stepnowsky C, et al. Sleep-disordered breathing in African-American elderly. Am J Respir Crit Care Med 1995;152:1946–9.

[35] Redline S, Tishler PV, Hans MG, et al. Racial differences in sleep-disordered breathing in African-Americans and Caucasians. Am J Respir Crit Care Med 1997;155:186–92.

[36] Kripke DF, Ancoli-Israel S, Klauber MR, et al. Prevalence of sleep-disordered breathing in ages 40–64 years: a population-based survey. Sleep 1997;20:65–76.

[37] Strohl KP, Saunders NA, Feldman NT, et al. Obstructive sleep apnea in family members. N Engl J Med 1978;299:969–73.

[38] Manon-Espaillat R, Gothe B, Adams N, et al. Familial 'sleep apnea plus' syndrome: report of a family. Neurology 1988;38:190–3.

[39] el Bayadi S, Millman RP, Tishler PV, et al. A family study of sleep apnea: anatomic and physiologic interactions. Chest 1990;98:554–9.

[40] Redline S, Tosteson T, Tishler PV, et al. Studies in the genetics of obstructive sleep apnea: familial aggregation of symptoms associated with sleep-related breathing disturbances. Am Rev Respir Dis 1992;145:440–4.

[41] Douglas NJ, Luke M, Mathur R. Is the sleep apnoea/hypopnoea syndrome inherited? Thorax 1993;48:719–21.

[42] Guilleminault C, Partinen M, Hollman K, et al. Familial aggregates in obstructive sleep apnea syndrome. Chest 1995;107:1545–51.

[43] Mathur R, Douglas NJ. Family studies in patients with the sleep apnea-hypopnea syndrome. Ann Intern Med 1995;122:174–8.

[44] Redline S, Tishler PV, Tosteson TD, et al. The familial aggregation of obstructive sleep apnea. Am J Respir Crit Care Med 1995;151:682–7.

[45] Schwab RJ, Gupta KB, Gefter WB, et al. Upper airway and soft tissue anatomy in normal subjects and patients with sleep-disordered breathing: significance of the lateral pharyngeal walls. Am J Respir Crit Care Med 1995;152:1673–89.

[46] Schwab RJ, Pasirstein M, Pierson R, et al. Identification of upper airway anatomic risk factors for obstructive sleep apnea with volumetric magnetic resonance imaging. Am J Respir Crit Care Med 2003;168:522–30.

[47] Schwartz AR, Smith PL, Wise RA, et al. Induction of upper airway occlusion in sleeping individuals with subatmospheric nasal pressure. J Appl Physiol 1988;64:535–42.

[48] Smith PL, Wise RA, Gold AR, et al. Upper airway pressure-flow relationships in obstructive sleep apnea. J Appl Physiol 1988;64:789–95.

[49] Suratt PM, McTier RF, Wilhoit SC. Upper airway muscle activation is augmented in patients with obstructive sleep apnea compared with that in normal subjects. Am Rev Respir Dis 1988;137:889–94.

[50] Mezzanotte WS, Tangel DJ, White DP. Waking genioglossal electromyogram in sleep apnea patients versus normal controls (a neuromuscular compensatory mechanism). J Clin Invest 1992;89:1571–9.

[51] Mezzanotte WS, Tangel DJ, White DP. Influence of sleep onset on upper-airway muscle activity in apnea patients versus normal controls. Am J Respir Crit Care Med 1996;153:1880–7.

[52] Vgontzas AN, Tan TL, Bixler EO, et al. Sleep apnea and sleep disruption in obese patients. Arch Intern Med 1994;154:1705–11.

[53] Smith PL, Gold AR, Meyers DA, et al. Weight loss in mildly to moderately obese patients with obstructive sleep apnea. Ann Intern Med 1985;103:850–5.

[54] Rubinstein I, Colapinto N, Rotstein LE, et al. Improvement in upper airway function after weight loss in patients with obstructive sleep apnea. Am Rev Respir Dis 1988;138:1192–5.

[55] Pasquali R, Colella P, Cirignotta F, et al. Treatment of obese patients with obstructive sleep apnea syndrome (OSAS): effect of weight loss and interference of otorhinolaryngoiatric pathology. Int J Obes 1990;14:207–17.

[56] Schwartz AR, Gold AR, Schubert N, et al. Effect of weight loss on upper airway collapsibility in obstructive sleep apnea. Am Rev Respir Dis 1991;144:494–8.

[57] Suratt PM, McTier RF, Findley LJ, et al. Effect of very-low-calorie diets with weight loss on obstructive sleep apnea. Am J Clin Nutr 1992;56(Suppl 1):S182–4.

[58] Kansanen M, Vanninen E, Tuunainen A, et al. The effect of a very low-calorie diet-induced weight loss on the severity of obstructive sleep apnoea and autonomic nervous function in obese patients with obstructive sleep apnoea syndrome. Clin Physiol Funct Imaging 1998;18: 377–85.

[59] Harman EM, Wynne JW, Block AJ. The effect of weight loss on sleep-disordered breathing and oxygen desaturation in morbidly obese men. Chest 1982;82:291–4.

[60] Peiser J, Lavie P, Ovnat A, et al. Sleep apnea syndrome in the morbidly obese as an indication for weight reduction surgery. Ann Surg 1984;199:112–5.

[61] Charuzi I, Ovnat A, Peiser J, et al. The effect of surgical weight reduction on sleep quality in obesity-related sleep apnea syndrome. Surgery 1985;97:535–8.

[62] Sugerman HJ, Fairman RP, Baron PL, et al. Gastric surgery for respiratory insufficiency of obesity. Chest 1986;90:81–6.

[63] Sharp JT, Henry JP, Sweany SK, et al. Effects of mass loading the respiratory system in man. J Appl Physiol 1964;19:959–66.

[64] Thut DC, Schwartz AR, Roach D, et al. Tracheal and neck position influence upper airway airflow dynamics by altering airway length. J Appl Physiol 1993;75:2084–90.

[65] Rowley JA, Permutt S, Willey S, et al. Effect of tracheal and tongue displacement on upper airway airflow dynamics. J Appl Physiol 1996;80:2171–8.

[66] Series F, Marc I. Influence of lung volume dependence of upper airway resistance during continuous negative airway pressure. J Appl Physiol 1994;77:840–4.

[67] Series F, Cormier Y, Desmeules M. Influence of passive changes of lung volume on upper airways. J Appl Physiol 1990;68:2159–64.

[68] Series F, Cormier Y, Couture J, Desmeules M. Changes in upper airway resistance with lung inflation and positive airway pressure. J Appl Physiol 1990;68:1075–9.

[69] Strohl KP, Redline S. Recognition of obstructive sleep apnea. Am J Respir Crit Care Med 1996; 154:279–89.

[70] Redline S. Epidemiology of sleep-disordered breathing. Respir Crit Care Med 1998;19:113–22.

[71] Brown IG, Zamel N, Hoffstein V. Pharyngeal cross-sectional area in normal men and women. J Appl Physiol 1986;61:890–5.

[72] Brooks LJ, Strohl KP. Size and mechanical properties of the pharynx in healthy men and women. Am Rev Respir Dis 1992;146:1394–7.

[73] Martin SE, Mathur R, Marshall I, et al. The effect of age, sex, obesity and posture an upper airway size. Eur Respir J 1997;10:2087–90.

[74] Schwab RJ, Gefter WB, Hoffman EA, et al. Dynamic upper airway imaging during awake respiration in normal subjects and patients with sleep disordered breathing. Am Rev Respir Dis 1993;148:1385–400.

[75] Whittle AT, Marshall I, Mortimore IL, et al. Neck soft tissue and fat distribution: comparison between normal men and women by magnetic resonance imaging. Thorax 1999;54:323–8.

[76] Pillar G, Malhotra A, Fogel R, et al. Airway mechanics and ventilation in response to resistive loading during sleep: influence of gender. Am J Respir Crit Care Med 2000;162:1627–32.

[77] Popovic RM, White DP. Upper airway muscle activity in normal women: influence of hormonal status. J Appl Physiol 1998;84:1055–62.

[78] Krystal AD, Edinger J, Wohlgemuth W, et al. Sleep in peri-menopausal and post-menopausal women. Sleep Med Rev 1998;2:243–53.

[79] Ancoli-Israel S, Kripke DF, Klauber MR, et al. Sleep-disordered breathing in community-dwelling elderly. Sleep 1991;14:486–95.

[80] Burger CD, Stanson AW, Sheedy PF, et al. Fast-computed tomography evaluation of age-related changes in upper airway structure and function in normal men. Am Rev Respir Dis 1992;145: 846–52.

[81] Hudgel DW, Devadatta P, Hamilton H. Pattern of breathing and upper airway mechanics during wakefulness and sleep in healthy elderly humans. J Appl Physiol 1993;74:2198–204.

[82] Martin SE, Mathur R, Marshall I, et al. The effect of age, sex, obesity and posture on upper airway size. Eur Respir J 1997;10:2087–90.

[83] Huang J, Shen H, Takahashi M, et al. Pharyngeal cross-sectional area and pharyngeal compliance in normal males and females. Respiration 1998;65:458–68.

[84] Kronenberg RS, Drage CW. Attenuation of the ventilatory and heart rate responses to hypoxia and hypercapnia with aging in normal men. J Clin Invest 1973;52:1812–9.

[85] Peterson DD, Pack AI, Silage DA, et al. Effects of aging on ventilatory and occlusion pressure responses to hypoxia and hypercapnia. Am Rev Respir Dis 1981;124:387–91.

[86] Brischetto MJ, Millman RP, Peterson DD, et al. Effect of aging on ventilatory response to exercise and CO2. J Appl Physiol 1984;56:1143–50.

[87] Naifeh KH, Severinghaus JW, Kamiya J, et al. Effect of aging on estimates of hypercapnic ventilatory response during sleep. J Appl Physiol 1989;66:1956–64.

[88] Worsnop C, Kay A, Kim Y, et al. Effect of age on sleep onset-related changes in respiratory pump and upper airway muscle function. J Appl Physiol 2000;88:1831–9.

[89] Ip MS, Lam B, Lauder IJ, et al. A community study of sleep-disordered breathing in middle-aged Chinese men in Hong Kong. Chest 2001;119:62–9.

[90] Ip MS, Lam B, Tang LC, et al. A community study of sleep-disordered breathing in middle-aged Chinese women in Hong Kong: prevalence and gender differences. Chest 2004;125:127–34.

[91] Li KK, Kushida C, Powell NB, et al. Obstructive sleep apnea syndrome: a comparison between Far-East Asian and white men. Laryngoscope 2000;110:1689–93.

[92] deBerry-Borowiecki B, Kukwa A, Blanks RH. Cephalometric analysis for diagnosis and treatment of obstructive sleep apnea. Laryngoscope 1988;98:226–34.

[93] Hochban W, Brandenburg U. Morphology of the viscerocranium in obstructive sleep apnoea syndrome: cephalometric evaluation of 400 patients. J Craniomaxillofac Surg 1994;22:205–13.

[94] Ferguson KA, Ono T, Lowe AA, et al. The relationship between obesity and craniofacial structure in obstructive sleep apnea. Chest 1995;108:375–81.

[95] Mayer P, Pepin JL, Bettega G, et al. Relationship between body mass index, age and upper airway measurements in snorers and sleep apnoea patients. Eur Respir J 1996;9:1801–9.

[96] Nelson S, Hans M. Contribution of craniofacial risk factors in increasing apneic activity among obese and nonobese habitual snorers. Chest 1997;111:154–62.

[97] Sakakibara H, Tong M, Matsushita K, et al. Cephalometric abnormalities in non-obese and obese patients with obstructive sleep apnoea. Eur Respir J 1999;13:403–10.

[98] Tangugsorn V, Krogstad O, Espeland L, et al. Obstructive sleep apnoea: multiple comparisons of cephalometric variables of obese and non-obese patients. J Craniomaxillofac Surg 2000; 28:204–12.

[99] Yu X, Fujimoto K, Urushibata K, et al. Cephalometric analysis in obese and nonobese patients with obstructive sleep apnea syndrome. Chest 2003;124:212–8.

[100] Sforza E, Bacon W, Weiss T, et al. Upper airway collapsibility and cephalometric variables in patients with obstructive sleep apnea. Am J Respir Crit Care Med 2000;161:347–52.

[101] Strohl KP, Saunders NA, Feldman NT, et al. Obstructive sleep apnea in family members. N Engl J Med 1978;299:969–73.

[102] Palmer LJ, Buxbaum SG, Larkin EK, et al. Whole genome scan for obstructive sleep apnea and obesity in African-American families. Am J Respir Crit Care Med 2004;169:1314–21.

[103] Palmer LJ, Buxbaum SG, Larkin E, et al. A whole-genome scan for obstructive sleep apnea and obesity. Am J Hum Genet 2003;72:340–50.

[104] Taasan VC, Block AJ, Boysen PG, et al. Alcohol increases sleep apnea and oxygen desaturation in asymptomatic men. Am J Med 1981;71:240–5.

[105] Block AJ, Hellard DW. Ingestion of either scotch or vodka induces equal effects on sleep and breathing of asymptomatic subjects. Arch Intern Med 1987;147:1145–7.

[106] Mitler MM, Dawson A, Henriksen SJ, et al. Bedtime ethanol increases resistance of upper airways and produces sleep apneas in asymptomatic snorers. Alcohol Clin Exp Res 1988;12: 801–5.

[107] Scrima L, Broudy M, Nay KN, et al. Increased severity of obstructive sleep apnea after bed-

time alcohol ingestion: diagnostic potential and proposed mechanism of action. Sleep 1982;5: 318–28.

[108] Scrima L, Hartman PG, Hiller FC. Effect of three alcohol doses on breathing during sleep in 30–49 year old nonobese snorers and nonsnorers. Alcohol Clin Exp Res 1989;13:420–7.

[109] Scanlan MF, Roebuck T, Little PJ, et al. Effect of moderate alcohol upon obstructive sleep apnoea. Eur Respir J 2000;16:909–13.

[110] Tsutsumi W, Miyazaki S, Itasaka Y, et al. Influence of alcohol on respiratory disturbance during sleep. Psychiatry Clin Neurosci 2000;54:332–3.

[111] Bonora M, Shields GI, Knuth SL, et al. Selective depression by ethanol of upper airway respiratory motor activity in cats. Am Rev Respir Dis 1984;130:156–61.

[112] Krol RC, Knuth SL, Bartlett Jr D. Selective reduction of genioglossal muscle activity by alcohol in normal human subjects. Am Rev Respir Dis 1984;129:247–50.

[113] Robinson RW, White DP, Zwillich CW. Moderate alcohol ingestion increases upper airway resistance in normal subjects. Am Rev Respir Dis 1985;132:1238–41.

ELSEVIER
SAUNDERS

Anesthesiology Clin N Am
23 (2005) 421–429

ANESTHESIOLOGY
CLINICS OF
NORTH AMERICA

Pathophysiologic Changes of Obesity

Kenneth F. Kuchta, MD

*Department of Anesthesiology, David Geffen School of Medicine at UCLA, Box 951778,
Los Angeles, CA 90095-1778, USA*

Obesity has recently taken the attention of the public media. Starting with a call to action by the Surgeon General, in 2001, to treat what was being labeled as an epidemic [1] to more recent concerns such as the increased fuel cost in commercial aviation resulting from obesity, [2,3] and whether the president is indeed overweight [4], a day rarely goes by without some news article related to the subject. Much of this recent emphasis can be traced to the extensive 1998 National Institutes of Health report on obesity [5,6]. This report provided extensive overviews of the available literature associating health risks with being overweight or obesity. Being overweight or obese is now a known risk factor for the development of diabetes, heart disease, stroke, hypertension, gallbladder disease, osteoarthritis, sleep apnea, other respiratory problems, and some forms of cancer (uterine, breast, colorectal, kidney, and gallbladder cancer). It is also associated with high serum cholesterol levels, complications of pregnancy, menstrual irregularities, hirsutism, stress incontinence, psychological disorders, and increased surgical risk. Not surprisingly, an increased mortality rate is associated with obesity [5,6].

The widespread dissemination of this information to the public and the health care community as well as the increased interest of these audiences in this subject are laudable from a public health perspective. For physicians, however, the emphasis should not stop with mere relationships and correlations. For our knowledge to truly increase, the mechanisms underlying these associations must be explored. Luckily, advances also are being made in our understanding of the pathophysiology of obesity. This article builds on the presently well-known changes that occur with obesity by drawing from recent advances reported in the literature for a better understanding of our obese patients.

E-mail address: kkuchta@mednet.ucla.edu

Cardiovascular pathophysiology

Recognition of the adverse implications of obesity for the cardiovascular system has been noted since Victorian times. The rigorous investigation of cardiac pathophysiology of obesity has occurred more recently. Early studies from the 1960s indicated that total blood volume and cardiac output were increased in obesity. Because heart rate remained unchanged, increased stroke volume was responsible for the change in cardiac output (CO). Regional blood flow in obese individuals was found to be similar to normal subjects, with the exception of splanchnic blood flow (slightly increased in obesity) and renal blood flow (slightly decreased). Oxygen consumption was found to increase in the obese, whereas systemic vascular resistance (SVR) decreased [7,8]. It could be argued that these findings represent mostly values uncorrected for body size. We would expect a 140-kg subject to have a higher cardiac output compared with a 70-kg control subject because the obese subject is perfusing more tissue. Because non-hypertensive obese patients do not show an increase in their mean arterial pressure (MAP) or a decrease in their central venous pressure (CVP) (the two factors in the numerator for the equation SVR = [MAP − CVP] ÷ CO), systemic vascular resistance must decrease. An alternate presentation of the cardiovascular parameters might include correction for the patient's size. This approach is also problematic because using body surface area (resulting in the cardiac index) results in values that are normal to subnormal, whereas using weight alone to correct results would be predicted to result in a significant drop in cardiac output (on a kilogram basis), compared with normal subjects. It is argued that this also obscures the increased absolute volume of blood that the cardiovascular system must deliver to the body in obesity [9]. Reframing this issue from a pathophysiologic perspective, the patient's cardiovascular system responds to the increased oxygen demand from the extra body tissue by increasing absolute blood volume, whereas the relative blood volume per kilogram decreases (from 86–47 mL/kg) [8]. This decrease might be expected because the added tissue would be mostly poorly perfused fat. The cardiovascular system still senses this as an increased oxygen demand that it meets by increasing cardiac output (through increased stroke volume because heart rate remains unchanged, as noted above).

Because the arterial venous oxygen difference is normal, this adaptation is successful, but there is good evidence that ventricular performance is impaired because the left ventricular stroke work index-to-left ventricular end diastolic pressure ratio is reduced and is negatively correlated with the degree of obesity. Increased stroke volume will result in increased end diastolic volume and pressure, which will result primarily in eccentric hypertrophy in the absence of hypertension. If the patient develops hypertension, a common comorbidity of obesity, concentric hypertrophy will develop along with an increase in SVR from low to normal or high levels compared with nonobese subjects. Either of these two mechanisms will result in increased left ventricular stroke work, whereas hypertension superimposed in obesity will act synergistically to dramatically increase the risk for cardiac failure [7–10].

Metabolic syndrome

A cluster of risk factors for the development of atherosclerotic cardiovascular disease was noted in diabetic patients in 1983. Originally named "syndrome X" in 1988 by Reaven [11], it has also been labeled variously as the multiple metabolic syndrome, insulin-resistance (IR) syndrome, the deadly quartet, and the dyslipidemia, IR, obesity, and high blood pressure (DROP) syndrome [11]. The World Health Organization (WHO) developed a working definition for what was then called the metabolic syndrome in 1999 [12]. The criteria for the diagnosis were further refined in 2001 by the National Cholesterol Education Program (NCEP) in its Adult Treatment Panel III [13]. In this latest incarnation, three risk factors must be present for the diagnosis of the metabolic syndrome. Abdominal obesity as measured by waist circumference (men $\geq$40 in and women $\geq$35 in) points to the frequently noted importance of android versus gynecoid obesity as it relates to the relative risk for the patient. Dyslipidemia is measured in two risk factors: a triglyceride level of more than 150 mg/dL and a high-density lipoprotein (HDL) cholesterol level less than 40 mg/dL in men and less than 50 mg/dL in women. Blood pressure higher than 130/$\geq$85 mm Hg and a fasting glucose level of more than 110 mg/dL are the last two risk factors [13]. The earlier WHO definition required only two risk factors and set slightly different limits, accepting a slightly higher blood pressure (up to 140/90) and slightly lower HDL level ($\leq$35 mg/dL in men and $\leq$39 mg/dL in women). The WHO criteria also include both impaired glucose regulation and insulin resistance as separate risk factors and microalbuminemia as another risk factor. Finally, an additional risk factor was listed, described as other conditional elements (such as hyperuricemia, coagulation disorders, or raised levels of plasminogen activator inhibitor-1) [12]. As noted above, insulin resistance is often considered a uniting force and part of the presumed pathophysiology linking the risk factors, even though its measurement or documentation is not required in the NCEP definition. The syndrome has also been associated with proinflammatory and hypercoagulable states [11,14].

Although a main purpose for defining the metabolic syndrome is to identify patients at risk, and to institute risk modification and indicated medical therapy, several implications for anesthesiologists also derive from work in this area. The diagnosis of obesity alone is less predictive for the development of diabetes, hypertension, renal failure, or atherosclerosis than the diagnosis of the metabolic syndrome [15]. An increased risk of at least twofold for atherosclerotic cardiovascular disease and a fivefold risk for type 2 diabetes have been found in patients with the metabolic syndrome [16]. For anesthesiologists, these increased risks would point to a subset of their obese patients who may be at increased operative risk. However, research in this area promises to contribute much more. It has been noted frequently that an abdominal distribution of obesity (android obesity) has more adverse physiologic consequences than a thigh and buttock distribution (gynecoid obesity). Although there is a debate as to whether these increased adverse consequences are the result of fat in the peritoneal cavity (omentum and mesentery) or in the subcutaneous tissue overlying the abdomen, in either case, abdominal distribution would be captured by some measure of abdominal girth (waist circumference or waist-to-hip measurement), and clearly its importance is being recognized in the criteria for the metabolic syndrome [16].

Perhaps the most exciting direction for the investigation and hypothesis coming from work related to the metabolic syndrome concerns a changing perspective about adipose tissue. Traditionally, adipose tissue has been considered a passive organ that merely stores energy; however, it is increasingly viewed as metabolically active, secreting hormone, cytokines, and other substances, with profound and far-reaching effects. The beginning of this change in thinking may be traced to the discovery of leptin, in 1994. This hormone, produced by adipose tissue, relays information about fat stores to the brain [15]. Leptin quickly captured the imagination of the press, with a photograph of a markedly obese mouse (the result of genetic mutations resulting in low leptin levels) placed next to a dramatically slimmer mouse with the same genetic defect, after being treated with leptin. The treatment resulted in reduced food intake, increased energy expenditure, and improvement in the rodent's diabetic condition [17]. The human version of leptin was licensed to Amgen (Thousand Oaks, CA). The initial fee of $20 million undoubtedly seemed insignificant compared with the prospect of a new wonder drug for dealing with the increasing epidemic of obesity. Humans with genetic mutations affecting leptin production have been identified, and as early as 1999, the reversal of obesity in a child with congenital leptin deficiency was reported [18].

Most obese patients are unlike either this patient or the laboratory model that contributed to her cure. Leptin levels tend to rise with weight, and most of the obese population tends to have genetically normal leptin and leptin receptors, as well as elevated leptin levels. The theory that the obese had become resistant to the effects of leptin and perhaps would benefit from even higher levels than produced endogenously was entertained. Early clinical trials were less than dramatic. Early subject dropout occurred because of injection-site redness and swelling. Significant weight loss occurred only in the two highest dose groups, with some of those subjects actually gaining weight [19–21]. It is clear that the physiology of leptin promises to be much more complex. Indeed, functional leptin receptors are found in many locations outside of the central nervous system, and it appears to have a role in organ systems ranging from reproduction to the immune system. It is this later association that may explain the proinflammatory tendency seen in the metabolic syndrome. An interesting theory speculates that the apparent resistance to the effects of leptin by the central nervous system in obesity may not be shared in other tissues of the body such as the immune system. Chronic leptin stimulation of the immune system (or other unmuted effects of elevated leptin) may result in the adverse cardiovascular effects of obesity. A high leptin level has been demonstrated to be an independent risk factor for adverse cardiac events in humans, and by comparison, those obese, leptin-deficient mice discussed above are resistant to atherosclerosis despite possessing other risk factors. As promising as this theory appears to be, it does not explain generally higher leptin levels found in women while demonstrating lower risk for cardiovascular disease. Clearly our understanding of the role of leptin in the pathophysiology of obesity is incomplete.

Another candidate for the mediation of feedback from adipose tissue for energy management and a proinflammatory signal is the cytokine interleukin (IL)-6. Unlike leptin, IL-6 is produced by both adipocytes and macrophages in fat. IL-6 levels seem most correlated with the level of obesity. Mice genetically deficient in IL-6 develop obesity, indicating the similarity with leptin. Several IL-6-related factors, including C-reactive protein, are probably intermediate mediators leading to arterial wall changes of atherosclerosis and chronic inflammation. IL-6 also causes increases in fibrinogen, platelet number, and platelet activity, contributing to clot formation [15].

Adipose tissue also releases an increased amount of nonesterified fatty acids (NEFAs), an amount beyond the body's energy needs. This occurs despite high levels of insulin, which normally suppress lipolysis. Excess NEFAs lead to a number of adverse outcomes, including the development of a fatty liver, insulin resistance, and an athrogenic dyslipidemia [16].

Other adipose tissue-derived mediators of inflammation have also been proposed, including tumor necrosis factor (TNF)-α, IL-1β, adiponectin, resistin, acylation-stimulating protein, serum amyloid A3 (SAA3), α1 acid glycoprotein, pentraxin-3, IL-1 receptor antagonist, and macrophage migration inhibitor factor. While these mediators may originate from a variety of cells (adipocytes, macrophages, or stromal cell) in adipose tissue, they all point to a much more metabolically active role than previously realized and offer exciting prospects for our further understanding of the pathophysiology of obesity [15].

Respiratory pathophysiology

Much like the cardiovascular system, a discussion of the respiratory pathophysiology of obesity begins with the metabolic demand imposed by the increased body mass from excess adipose tissue. This demand is further complicated by the increased work of breathing caused by reduced respiratory system compliance resulting from fat in the abdominal cavity as well as in and around the chest wall and diaphragm. Reduced lung volumes may contribute to this pathology by increasing respiratory resistance. Respiratory muscle dysfunction also has been reported with obesity [22] and may result from an inefficiency secondary to changes in chest wall compliance or the lower lung volumes found in obesity. Reported decreases in maximum voluntary ventilation (MVV) may indicate concomitantly decreased respiratory muscle endurance [23]. The toll for the respiratory system can be measured in increased oxygen consumption (VO_2) and carbon dioxide production even at rest. This reaction occurs in a setting of the disproportionately higher proportion of VO_2 required for respiration even during quiet breathing. As a result, minute ventilation is increased even at rest. In obesity, lung volumes are altered, with decreased functional residual capacity

(FRC), in which diminished expiratory reserve volume accounts for the change, as reserve volume remains unchanged. Total lung capacity (TLC) and vital capacity (VC) may be reduced. A ventilation-perfusion mismatch caused by lung closure within the range of VC in obesity results in hypoxia. Forced expiratory volume in one second (FEV_1) is decreased but appears to be proportionate to decreases in forced vital capacity (FVC) resulting in no changes in the FEV_1-FVC ratio. In those patients with upper-body obesity (android obesity), more marked decreases in FVC, FEV_1, and TLC are reported. Weight loss in the obese patient is associated with an improvement in FRC, VC, TLC, and MVV.

The obesity-hypoventilation syndrome (OHS), an extreme disorder seen in some obese patients, was described in 1955 and labeled the Pickwickian syndrome in 1956, because these patients seemed to resemble an obese character (the messenger boy Joe) in Charles Dickens' "The Pickwick Papers." The disorder is characterized by alveolar hypoventilation, chronic hypercapnia and hypoxia, hypersomnolence, polycythemia, and right ventricular failure. Other factors beyond obesity must be part of the pathophysiology of OHS because body weight alone does not correlate with daytime hypercapnia. The "normal" response to hypercapnia and hypoxia, increased minute ventilation, is enhanced in obese patients not suffering from OHS. A relationship with obstructive sleep apnea (OSA) is suggested, but the exact relationship is far from clear. These facts not withstanding, weight loss can reverse the hypercapnia found in OHS.

There is some epidemiologic evidence for an association between obesity and asthma and the tendency for obesity to precede asthma in some patients. Certainly, small airway collapse seen with decreased lung volumes and the shallow breathing found in the obese could contribute to asthma because both breathing patterns and airway diameter may have an impact on airway responsiveness. Chronic inflammation appears to be a common feature in both asthma and obesity. This line of thinking has led to the speculation that mediators such as IL-6 or cyclooxygenase-2 from adipose tissue might contribute to asthma in the obese patient. Even the reduced intake of antioxidants has been suggested to explain the obesity-asthma association. Gastroesophageal reflux also might be part of the link because its incidence is higher in obesity, and reflux has been associated with asthma [22].

The role of a more metabolically active adipose tissue (the adipose endocrinology) has been alluded to in the relationship between asthma and obesity. Leptin appears to have a role in respiratory pathophysiology. Genetically obese leptin-deficient mice also suffer from respiratory depression and altered respiratory mechanics. These animals also were found to have an altered response to carbon dioxide and hypercapnia, which is a characteristic of OHS. Replacing leptin in these animals dramatically increased their minute ventilation. Although it was difficult to control for concomitant weight loss when treating these animals, it appears that leptin had a role in regulating central respiration as well as acting as a growth factor in lung. As noted, most human obesity is associated with high leptin levels and a possible leptin resistance with regard to energy metabolism. It is speculated that a similar mechanism, a relative resistance to the respiratory effects of leptin, may be operating in OHS or OSA [24]. More recently, it has been observed that leptin levels are increased during sleep and decreased with sleep deprivation. This observation has led to the speculation that leptin may be a link in a complex pathway among chronic sleep loss, sleep-disordered breathing (such as OSA), obesity, and the metabolic syndrome [25]. Once again, there is evidence of leptin and other products of adipose tissue interacting with a variety of organ systems and body functions in complicated ways that are only beginning to be understood.

Cancer

Obesity has been demonstrated to increase the risk for a variety of carcinomas including colon, breast, endometrial, renal, gallbladder, and esophageal cancer [26], a relationship that points to an additional large health risk for the obese population. It has been suggested that overeating is the largest "avoidable" cancer risk in nonsmokers. If the relationship is truly causal, being overweight and obese are causes of cancer death in 1 of 7 males and 1 of 5 females [27]. Our recent understanding of the pathophysiology of cancer in obesity has begun to increase dramatically. For esophageal cancer, the risk seems to be related to an increased incidence of gastroesophageal reflux and the development of Barrett's esophagus. A number of theories have been proposed to explain the remaining increased cancer risks, but in humans, the mechanism with the most supporting evidence centers around the alteration of endogenous hormone metabolism, mainly androgens, estrogen, progesterone, and insulin [28]. Increased levels of insulin indirectly result in increased levels of free insulin-like growth factor (ILGF)-1 by decreasing the amount of their binding protein (ILGFBP-1 and ILGFBP-2). This increase in free ILGF-1 may be significant in that it stimulates cell proliferation and decreases apoptosis and is a strong mitogen for several cancers. Insulin also inhibits the production of sex hormone-binding globulin by the liver. The resultant increased free sex hormones can be further enhanced by adipocyte conversion of androgens to estrogen. These effects on sex hormones can affect some cancers [27]. This is one more example of a much more active metabolic role for adipose tissue than previously suspected, especially with regard to hyperinsulinemia, with pathophysiologic consequences that we are only beginning to understand and that range far beyond our original conception of inert adipose tissue.

Summary

The medical community and the public are becoming increasingly aware of the profound impact that obesity has on health. The impact of obesity ranges over a variety of organ systems, with a large number of risk factors for significant disease. Dramatic increases in our understanding of the pathophysiology of obesity have resulted from the realization that adipose tissue, in addition to being a burden with respect to increased weight and oxygen consumption, is more metabolically active than suspected previously. The end products of this metabolism, especially hormones, cytokines, and proinflammatory mediators, have far ranging affects with important health consequences.

References

[1] US Department of Health and Human Services. The Surgeon General's call to action to prevent and decrease overweight and obesity. Rockville, MD: US DHHS, Public Health Service, Office of the Surgeon General; 2001. Available at: http://www.surgeongeneral.gov/library. Accessed January 1, 2005.

[2] Feds: obesity raising airline fuel costs. USA Today Web site. November 5, 2004 [updated Nov 7, 2004]. Available at: http://www.usatoday.com/travel/news/2004-11-05-obese-fliers_x.htm. Accessed January 1, 2005.

[3] Dannenberg AL, Burton DC, Jackson RJ. Economic and environmental costs of obesity. Am J Prev Med 2004;27(3):264.

[4] Kolata G. Tell the truth: does this index make me look fat? The New York Times. November 28, 2004;sect4:6.

[5] National Institutes of Health, National Heart, Lung and Blood Institute. Clinical guidelines on the identification, evaluation, and treatment of overweight and obesity in adults. DHHS, Public Health Service; 1998 [NIH Publication No. 98–4083]. Available at: http://www.nhlbi. nih.gov/guidelines/obesity/ob_home.htm. Accessed January 1, 2005.

[6] WIN Statistics page. The Weight-control Information Network website. Available at: http://win. niddk.nih.gov/statistics/index.htm. Accessed January 1, 2005.

[7] Alpert MA, Hashimi MW. Obesity and the heart. Am J Med Sci 1993;306(2):117–23.

[8] Alexander JK, Dennis EW, Smith WG, et al. Blood volume, cardiac output, and distribution of systemic blood flow in extreme obesity. Cardiovascular Research Center Bulletin 1962–1963; 1(2):39–44.

[9] Messerli FH. Cardiovascular effects of obesity and hypertension. Lancet 1982;1(8282):1165–8.

[10] de Divitiis O, Fazio S, Petitto M, et al. Obesity and cardiac function. Circulation 1981;64(3): 477–82.

[11] Scott CL. Diagnosis, prevention, and intervention for the metabolic syndrome. Am J Cardiol 2003;92(Suppl i):S35–42.

[12] Definition, diagnosis and classification of diabetes mellitus and its complications. Part 1: diagnosis and classification of diabetes mellitus. Geneva: World Health Organization, Department of Noncommunicable Disease Surveillance; 1999. p. 31–3.

[13] Expert Panel on Detection. Evaluation, and treatment of high blood cholesterol in adults: executive summary of the third report of the national cholesterol education program (NCEP) expert panel on detection, evaluation, and treatment of high blood cholesterol in adults (Adult Treatment Panel III). JAMA 2001;285(19):2486–97.

[14] Vaga GL. Cardiovascular outcomes for obesity and metabolic syndrome. Obes Res 2002; 10(Suppl 1):S27–32.

[15] Wisse BE. The inflammatory syndrome: the role of adipose tissue cytokines in metabolic disorders linked to obesity. J Am Soc Nephrol 2004;15(11):2792–800.

[16] Grundy SM. Obesity, metabolic syndrome, and cardiovascular disease. J Clin Endocrinol Metab 2004;89(6):2595–600.

[17] Body weight regulated by newly discovered hormone [July 27, 1995; updated April 7, 1998]. The Rockefeller University Web site. Available at: http://www.rockefeller.edu/pubinfo/ob.rel. nr.html. Accessed January 1, 2005.

[18] Farooqi IS, Jebb SA, Langmack G, et al. Effects of recombinant leptin therapy in a child with congenital leptin deficiency. N Engl J Med 1999;341(12):879–84.

[19] Gura T. Leptin not impressive in clinical trial. Science 1999;286(5441):881–2.

[20] Yanovski JA, Yanovski SZ. Recent advances in basic obesity research. JAMA 1999;282(16): 1504–6.

[21] Heymsfield SB, Greenberg AS, Fujioka K, et al. Recombinant leptin for weight control in obese and lean adults. JAMA 1999;282(16):1568–75.

[22] Jubber AS. Respiratory complications of obesity. Int J Clin Pract 2004;58(6):573–80.

[23] Weiner P, Waizman J, Weiner M, et al. Influence of excessive weight loss after gastroplasty for morbid obesity on respiratory muscle performance. Thorax 1998;53(1):39–42.

[24] O'Donnell CP, Tankersley CG, Polotsky VP, et al. Leptin, obesity, and respiratory function. Respir Physiol 2000;119:173–80.

[25] Saaresranta T, Olli P. Does leptin link sleep loss and breathing disturbances with major public diseases? Ann Med 2004;36(3):172–83.

[26] Calle EE, Rodriguez C, Walker-Thurmond K, et al. Overweight, obesity, and mortality from cancer in a prospectively studied cohort of US adults. N Engl J Med 2003;348(17):1625–38.

[27] Calle EE, Thun MJ. Obesity and cancer. Oncogene 2004;23(38):6365–78.

[28] Bianchini F, Kaaks R, Vainio H. Overweight, obesity, and cancer risk. Lancet Oncol 2002;3(9): 565–74.

ELSEVIER
SAUNDERS

Anesthesiology Clin N Am
23 (2005) 431–443

ANESTHESIOLOGY
CLINICS OF
NORTH AMERICA

Pathophysiology of Obstructive Sleep Apnea

Annette G. Pashayan, MD*, Anthony N. Passannante, MD, Peter Rock, MD, MBA, FCCP, FCCM

Department of Anesthesiology, University of North Carolina School of Medicine, N2201, CB 7010, Chapel Hill, NC 27599-7010, USA

Sleep apnea is a general term encompassing two distinct entities, central sleep apnea and obstructive sleep apnea (OSA). Central sleep apnea is a relatively uncommon disorder caused by abnormal neurologic control of the diaphragm, resulting in the loss of respiratory effort. OSA, on the other hand, is much more common and affects more than 10% of the population over 65 years of age and men more often than women [1–3]. OSA involves episodic collapse and blockage of the upper airway during sleep despite continuous respiratory effort. This article explores the physiologic basis and symptoms of OSA.

Obstructive disruption of breathing during sleep can be divided into three categories: OSA, obstructive sleep hypopnea, and upper airway resistance [4]. Fig. 1 shows the distinctive physiologic characteristics of each category in the form of data obtained during sleep studies. The sleep study, or polysomnogram, is a comprehensive battery of physiologic measurements taken in a sleep laboratory, used to diagnose a variety of sleep disorders. "Obstructive apnea" is defined as the total cessation of airflow for 10 seconds or more despite continued ventilatory effort. Patients suffering five or more such apneas per hour of sleep are considered to have OSA. Apneic episodes are usually associated with a decrease in oxyhemoglobin saturation of 4% or more. "Obstructive sleep hypopnea," on the other hand, is defined as a decrease of 30% to 50% in airflow for 10 seconds or longer. Hypopnea may also be associated with the desaturation of oxyhemo-

---

* Corresponding author.
E-mail address: apashayan@aims.unc.edu (A.G. Pashayan).

0889-8537/05/$ – see front matter © 2005 Elsevier Inc. All rights reserved.
doi:10.1016/j.atc.2005.02.004
anesthesiology.theclinics.com

globin. "Upper airway resistance" is characterized by snoring during sleep without frank apnea or hypopnea and therefore does not result in oxyhemoglobin desaturation. Many sleep study laboratories report polysomnographic data as the combined number of apneic and hypopnic episodes per hour of sleep, the apnea-hypopnea index (AHI).

All three types of sleep obstructive breathing, apnea, hypopnea, and airway resistance, are associated with respiratory-related arousals from sleep. Following the arousal, the sleeper reinitiates ventilation and then tries to resume

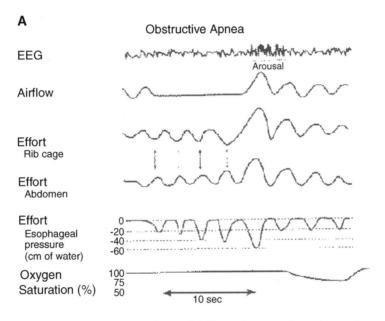

Fig. 1. Manifestations of upper airway closure. (*A*) Obstructive apnea. Increasing ventilatory effort is seen in the rib cage, the abdomen, and the level of esophageal pressure (measured with an esophageal balloon), despite the lack of oronasal airflow. Arousal on the electroencephalogram (EEG) is associated with increasing ventilatory effort, as indicated by the esophageal pressure. Oxy-hemoglobin desaturation follows the termination of apnea. Note that during apnea, the movements of the rib cage and the abdomen (Effort) are in opposite directions (*arrows*) as a result of attempts to breathe against a closed airway. Once the airway opens in response to arousal, rib cage and abdominal movements become synchronous. (*B*) Obstructive hypopnea. Decreased airflow is associated with increasing ventilatory effort (reflected by the esophageal pressure) and subsequent arousal on the EEG. Rib cage and abdominal movements are in opposite directions during hypopnea (*arrows*), reflecting increasingly difficult breathing against a partially closed airway. Rib cage and abdominal movements become synchronous after arousal, producing airway opening. Oxyhemoglobin desaturation follows the termination of hypopnea. (*C*) Upper airway resistance. Asynchronous movements of the rib cage and abdomen and a substantial decrease in airflow are not seen. Arousal observed on the EEG is associated with increasing ventilatory effort because of increased airway resistance, as reflected by the esophageal pressure. There is no significant oxyhemoglobin desaturation. (*From* Strollo Jr PJ, Rogers RM. Obstructive sleep apnea. N Engl J Med 1996;334:99–104; with permission.)

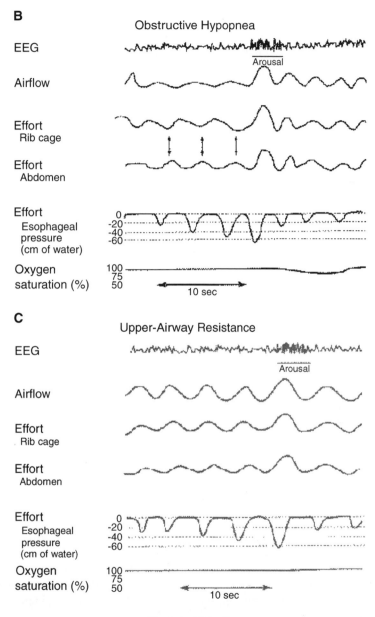

Fig. 1 (*continued*).

sleep. Sleep fragmentation results in excessive daytime sleepiness (EDS) and after time may lead to long-term neurocognitive, metabolic, and cardiovascular problems. The occurrence of an AHI greater than 5 in combination with symptoms of hypersomnolence meets the diagnostic criteria for sleep apnea syndrome [2].

Cause of obstructive sleep apnea

Airflow obstruction in OSA may occur at any point in the upper airway from the soft palate to the hypopharynx posterior to the tongue [5]. The patency of the normal upper airway is determined by pharyngeal transmural pressure, defined as the difference between the pressure within the airway lumen and the pressure exerted by tissues surrounding the site of collapse. Recent findings [6] suggest that a decrease in pharyngeal transmural pressure alone is a sufficient condition for the production of OSA syndrome in normal individuals.

During spontaneous inspiration, contraction of the diaphragm results in sub-atmospheric pressure throughout the airway, promoting airflow into the respiratory tract. In the face of negative intraluminal pressure, the lower airway normally remains patent because of the structural support of circumferential cartilaginous rings in the tracheobronchial tree. The upper airway lacks such support and is dependent on the malleable configuration of soft tissue. Upper airway patency is therefore vulnerable to various influences such as muscle tone, tissue mass, and tissue consistency. The loss of forces that maintain soft tissue structural integrity contributes significantly to airway obstruction in OSA. Pharyngeal muscle tone decreases during stage 4 and rapid eye movement sleep [7,8], resulting in some degree of upper airway narrowing even in normal sleeping individuals. Various other structural factors such as obesity, macroglossia, and enlarged tonsils may further narrow the pharyngeal lumen and increase the likelihood of airway collapse during inspiration [9,10].

Gravity plays an important role in the obstruction of breathing during sleep [11,12]. Sleep studies performed on astronauts have found a significantly lower incidence of apnea, hypopnea, and snoring during space flight than on earth [12]. In the presence of gravity, changing from a supine to a lateral position improves the ability of the airway to remain patent during negative pressures [11] by enlarging retropalatal and retroglossal aspects of the airway.

The Pickwickian syndrome is a severe form of OSA seen in morbidly obese individuals with right heart failure. Although patients need not be obese to develop OSA, and not all obese individuals have sleep apnea, patients with a body mass index greater than 35 are at greater risk for OSA. Patients suffering from OSA are often fatigued, which may lead to inactivity and subsequent obesity. Obese individuals are also likely to have redundant airway tissue, which exacerbates airway obstruction. Weight loss is indicated for the initial management of OSA, particularly in overweight individuals, and often leads to improvement in the disease.

Sleep-disordered breathing is common in the middle-aged population [1–3]: 9% of women and 24% of men have an AHI of 5 or more, and 2% of women and 4% of men suffer from sleep apnea syndrome [2]. OSA is therefore a significant public health problem [13,14], much like diabetes mellitus or asthma. An increased incidence of OSA has been found in certain groups. For example, commercial truck drivers have a 46% incidence of OSA, and professional football players have a 14% incidence of OSA [15,16]. Individuals with OSA have a significantly higher mortality rate compared with those without the disease, perhaps as much as a sevenfold increase [17,18], and it is estimated that OSA contributes to the deaths of approximately 40,000 Americans per year [18].

Contributing factors

Abnormalities in the autonomic control of the pharyngeal muscles may contribute to airway obstruction, perhaps by changing the balance between forces promoting the patency of the airway and those favoring its collapse [19]. An intriguing study [20] of OSA patients with permanent atrial pacemakers found that subjects had fewer episodes of OSA if their pacemakers were set to increase their heart rate during the night. It is hypothesized that the increased vagal tone accompanying bradycardia also affects airway patency. Another study series [21] of patients undergoing ECG Holter monitoring showed that nocturnal paroxysmal asystole, episodic bradycardia, and sinus node dysfunction were more prevalent in patients with OSA. Autonomic dysfunction and OSA have been linked in other studies [22,23], but a cause and effect relationship is not yet clear. It has been postulated [24] that autonomic chemoreceptors reacting to hypoxia, hypercapnia, and acidosis trigger an inflammatory cascade with numerous downstream consequences including hypertension, insulin resistance, atherosclerosis, and metabolic syndrome.

The preponderance of males with OSA points to gonadal hormones as a potential influence in the development and severity of OSA. A randomized placebo-controlled study [25] in which healthy elderly men received variable amounts of intramuscular testosterone demonstrated shortened sleep, worsened sleep apnea, and increased duration of hypoxemia with testosterone treatment. Studies of androgen deprivation [26,27], however, have shown little or no change in sleep or breathing. This supports an "estrogen protection" hypothesis and is consistent with studies of women in whom OSA increased after menopause and was improved with hormone replacement therapy [28–30].

Individuals with specific endocrine diseases, namely acromegaly, Cushing's syndrome, hypothyroidism, and diabetes mellitus, are at higher risk for OSA [31]. The hormonal imbalances in these disorders lead to structural distortion of the airway, predisposing to obstruction. In acromegaly, in which the frequency of OSA is as high as 60%, an excess of growth hormone produces craniofacial changes that are thought to be pathogenic [32]. Fig. 2 illustrates the specific craniofacial changes that can occur in acromegaly leading to airway obstruction. The high incidence of OSA in Cushinoid patients is attributed largely to weight gain, particularly adipose accumulation in parapharyngeal spaces [33]. In the case of hypothyroidism, low thyroid hormone alone has not been shown to cause OSA unless myxedema is present, resulting in edema and myopathy [31]. In noninsulin-dependent type 2 diabetes mellitus, obesity is a common risk factor for both OSA and insulin resistance, and OSA may actually contribute to the

A   B

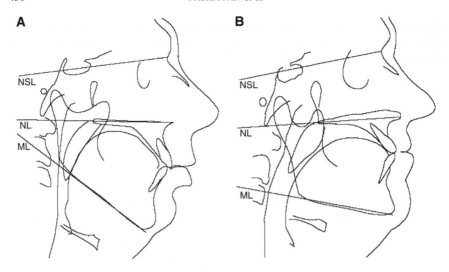

Fig. 2. Example of an acromegalic patient with (*A*) and without (*B*) OSA. Note the vertical facial growth with steep mandibular line (ML, from inferior point of bony chin [menton] to a mid-planed point at the gonial angle) and pharyngeal narrowing (*A*) as apposed to horizontal facial growth with flat ML and no pharyngeal narrowing (*B*). NL, nasal line, through the most anterior point of anterior nasal spine and most posterior point of hard palate; NSL, nasal-sella line, from nasion to sella. (*From* Hochban W, Ehlenz K, Conradt R, et al. Obstructive sleep apnoea in acromegaly: the role of craniofacial changes. Eur Respir J 1999;14:196–202; with permission.)

development of type 2 diabetes [31]. In insulin-dependent type 1 diabetes mellitus, autonomic neuropathy may contribute to development of OSA [34].

Airway moisture and surface tension in the fluid lining the upper airway also play a role in maintaining airway patency [35,36]. A reduction of surface tension in the pharyngeal lining fluid by the instillation of a surfactant correlates with a decrease in upper airway collapsibility and a lessening of sleep apnea severity as measured by AHI. It has been postulated [37] that continuous snoring and the impairment of airflow during sleep dry the pharyngeal mucosa and elevates surface tension. Increasing surface tension leads to worse airflow obstruction and mucosal trauma and thus increases the severity of sleep apnea. Furthermore, dry mucosa may alter the function of pharyngeal sensory receptors, further impairing airway patency.

Obstructive sleep apnea symptoms

As mentioned previously, three distinct patterns of sleep-disordered breathing have been defined as apnea, hypopnea, and upper airway resistance (see Fig. 1). There is considerable disagreement in the literature as to whether these three patterns represent distinct syndromes, different manifestations of one syndrome, or stages in the development of a single syndrome [4,10]. However, all three patterns of sleep-obstructed breathing result in an increased ventilatory effort in response to airway closure, with subsequent arousal, sleep fragmentation, and EDS.

Box 1 lists symptoms of OSA, the most common of which are snoring, EDS, and sudden arousals with choking [38]. Snoring occurs in almost all patients with OSA, but because snoring is so common in the general population, it is, by itself, a poor predictor of OSA. However, the absence of snoring makes a diagnosis of OSA unlikely, because less than 6% of patients with OSA are not reported to snore [39]. A history of snoring elicited on a preoperative history is therefore a useful predictor of a patient's tendency toward airway obstruction in the perioperative period.

Individuals with OSA experience cycles of sleep, obstruction, arousal, restoration of breathing, and falling asleep again, and they may suffer dozens of such cycles in an hour. This cycle results in poor sleep quality and EDS. Patients with OSA may fall asleep at work or while driving or operating machinery and have an increased number of work and car accidents [40–42].

Nocturnal choking and apnea are the third most common complaints of patients diagnosed with OSA. Bed partners may witness pauses in breathing, and the patients themselves may report waking up in a state of acute panic. Such episodes may be brief in duration, but they are of considerable concern to patients and their bed partners [38]. In addition to the above symptoms, OSA patients report other problems, including headaches [43], depression, impotence, and enuresis (see Box 1).

Box 1. Symptoms of obstructive sleep apnea

Snoring*
Excessive daytime sleepiness*
Sudden arousals with choking*
Unrefreshing sleep
Fatigue
Lethargy
Depression
Morning dry throat
Morning headaches
Impotence
Enuresis
Nocturnal sweating

* Most common presenting symptoms of OSA

Diseases associated with obstructive sleep apnea

Patients with OSA frequently display various comorbidities (Box 2). Although it is not established whether these conditions are the result or the cause of OSA, it is reasonable to postulate that the associated comorbidities derive, at least in part, from the pathophysiologic consequences of sleep-obstructed breathing.

There is extensive epidemiologic evidence linking OSA to systemic hypertension, even in the absence of obesity [44–46]. The episodes of oxyhemoglobin desaturation and arousal seen in OSA are accompanied by the activation of the sympathetic nervous system. This results in direct vasoconstriction and the subsequent stimulation of the renin-angiotensin-aldosterone system (RAAS) [47]. The relationship among obesity, sleep apnea, and the activation of various components of the RAAS is complex. Studies [48] have shown elevated plasma levels of both angiotensin II and aldosterone in patients with OSA, but the treatment of OSA with continuous positive airway pressure (CPAP) did not significantly lower these hormones and lowered blood pressure only modestly. Also contributing to the development of hypertension in OSA patients is a reduction of circulating levels of nitric oxide, which have been shown to increase after CPAP treatment [49].

As mentioned previously, OSA is commonly associated with obesity. Obese patients are at a greater risk for airway obstruction resulting from increased fat deposits in parapharyngeal tissues. Obese patients with OSA and EDS tend to become sedentary, which further contributes to obesity. Thus, a vicious cycle is set up whereby obesity contributes to OSA and vice versa.

Sleep apnea is common in diabetic individuals, and there are some data that suggest that OSA contributes to the development of glucose intolerance. A study [50] of men suspected of having OSA who underwent sleep studies and glucose tolerance tests found that the AHI is an independent predictor of blood glucose levels and insulin sensitivity and that type 2 diabetes occurs with a high frequency in OSA. A study [51] of premenopausal women showed a 30-fold increase in sleep-disordered breathing in subjects with insulin resistance secondary

---

Box 2. Comorbidities associated with obstructive sleep apnea

Hypertension
Obesity
Diabetes mellitus
Coronary artery disease
Cerebral vascular disease and stroke
Congestive heart failure
Cardiac dysrhythmias
Gastroesophageal reflux disease

to polycystic ovary syndrome compared with control subjects. Two published studies [52,53] report improvement in insulin sensitivity with CPAP treatment of OSA, again supporting the notion that OSA and insulin sensitivity are linked directly. It has been postulated that hypoxemia produced during airway obstruction alters adrenergic function, thus affecting glucose metabolism both directly and by way of inflammatory intermediates [54]. Still, other authors [55] state that the relationship between OSA and insulin resistance is mediated primarily by their common factor, obesity.

OSA is a risk factor for first and recurrent stroke and post-stroke mortality [56]. Stroke victims are known to suffer sleep-disordered breathing and to be at risk for both central and obstructive apneas during the acute phase of their stroke. During recovery from stroke, central apneas decline in occurrence, but OSA frequently continues [57]. OSA is a more common long-term consequence of ischemic stroke than of hemorrhagic stroke [58]. During obstructive apneas, cerebral blood flow velocity temporarily increases, with a subsequent decrease after apnea termination. The changes in cerebral blood flow velocity are accompanied by parallel changes in blood pressure. It is postulated that low cerebral blood flow velocity and low blood pressure along with hypoxemia immediately following apneic spells contribute to the development of ischemic stroke [57]. Additionally, OSA patients have a high incidence of atherosclerosis, which also contributes to ischemic stroke.

There is a strong correlation between OSA and atherosclerotic cardiovascular disease. Although the pathophysiology is complex and poorly understood [59,60], several lines of evidence suggest that vascular endothelial function may be altered in OSA individuals, predisposing them to atherosclerosis. A recent large study [61] showed that the AHI and the percentage of time below 90% oxygen saturation were associated with endothelial dysfunction as determined by impaired brachial artery flow-mediated dilation. Patients with OSA have shown an attenuated response to vasodilators [62] as well as functional down-regulation of vascular α- and β-adrenergic receptors [63]. OSA is associated with an increased expression of adhesion molecules on monocytes, an increased adherence of monocytes to human endothelial cells in culture, and an increased production of reactive oxygen species [64]. Finally, increased platelet activation and aggregation occur during sleep in patients with OSA [65].

Repeated activation of the sympathetic nervous system and changes in vagal tone in response to oxyhemoglobin desaturation may also play a role in the development and worsening of pre-existing coronary artery disease. Although OSA patients have been shown to develop myocardial ischemia during sleep, there is only a poor temporal association between periods of apnea and episodes of myocardial ischemia [66]. Mechanisms for myocardial ischemia in this context include activation of the sympathetic nervous system with increased cardiac afterload, increased myocardial work, and increased oxygen demand. The increased oxygen demand occurs in a setting of reduced oxygen delivery caused by oxyhemoglobin desaturation. Myocardial oxygen supply may be further impaired by anemia in postoperative patients.

Sleep-disordered breathing is common in patients with congestive heart failure [67], and diastolic heart dysfunction appears to be associated with a significantly increased risk of OSA [68]. The Framingham Heart Study [69] found echocardiographic evidence of right ventricular hypertrophy in subjects with sleep-disordered breathing. OSA patients are also predisposed to clinically significant cardiac dysrhythmias [21], which can be controlled with CPAP [70]. There is a high prevalence of OSA in patients with reduced left ventricular ejection fraction who require an implantable cardioverter-defibrillator for severe dysrhythmias [71].

A link between OSA and gastroesophageal reflux disease (GERD) has been suggested [72–74], and CPAP has been shown to decrease GERD symptoms in OSA patients [75]. However, there are no data to suggest that GERD causes airway obstruction or that OSA is causative in the development of GERD [76–78].

Summary

OSA, a common disease among middle aged men and to a lesser degree in postmenopausal women, results from episodic upper airway obstruction during sleep. Episodes of airway obstruction cause arousal and sleep fragmentation, which result in EDS. This disorder is associated with various other diseases, including hypertension, diabetes mellitus, atherosclerotic heart disease, cerebrovascular disease, and gastroesophageal reflux disease. The fact that all these disorders are, like OSA, more common in cases of obesity makes it difficult to determine the exact progression of pathophysiologic events, but a growing body of evidence suggests that OSA is an independent factor in the development of serious morbidity.

References

[1] Drazen JM. Sleep apnea syndrome. N Engl J Med 2002;346:390.
[2] Young T, Palta M, Dempsey J, et al. The occurrence of sleep-disordered breathing among middle-aged adults. N Engl J Med 1993;328:1230–5.
[3] Collop NA. The significance of sleep-disordered breathing and obstructive sleep apnea in the elderly. Chest 1997;112:867–8.
[4] Strollo Jr PJ, Rogers RM. Obstructive sleep apnea. N Engl J Med 1996;334:99–104.
[5] Hudgel DW. Variable site of airway narrowing among obstructive sleep apnea patients. J Appl Physiol 1986;61:1403–9.
[6] King ED, O'Donnell CP, Smith PL, et al. A model of obstructive sleep apnea in normal humans. Role of the upper airway. Am J Respir Crit Care Med 2000;161:1979–84.
[7] Benumof JL. Obstructive sleep apnea in the adult obese patient: implications for airway management. J Clin Anesth 2001;13:144–56.
[8] Loadsman JA, Wilcox I. Is obstructive sleep apnoea a rapid eye movement-predominant phenomenon? Br J Anaesth 2000;85:354–8.
[9] Badr MS, Zahn BR. Images in clinical medicine: upper-airway resistance syndrome. N Engl J Med 2000;342:1408.

[10] Guilleminault C, Chowdhuri S. Upper airway resistance syndrome is a distinct syndrome. Am J Respir Crit Care Med 2000;161:1412–3.

[11] Isono S, Tanaka A, Nishino T. Lateral position decreases collapsibility of the passive pharynx in patients with obstructive sleep apnea. Anesthesiology 2002;97:780–5.

[12] Elliott AR, Shea SA, Dijk DJ, et al. Microgravity reduces sleep-disordered breathing in humans. Am J Respir Crit Care Med 2001;164:478–85.

[13] Phillipson EA. Sleep apnea–a major public health problem. N Engl J Med 1993;328:1271–3.

[14] National health interview survey. Available at: http://www.pop.psu.edu./data-archive/daman/nhis1.htm.

[15] George CF, Kab V, Levy AM. Increased prevalence of sleep-disordered breathing among professional football players. N Engl J Med 2003;348:367–8.

[16] Stoohs RA, Bingham LA, Itoi A, et al. Sleep and sleep-disordered breathing in commercial long-haul truck drivers. Chest 1995;107:1275–82.

[17] National Commission on Sleep Disorders Research. Wake up America: a national sleep alert. Washington, DC: Government Printing Office; 1993.

[18] He J, Kryger MH, Zorick FJ, et al. Mortality and apnea index in obstructive sleep apnea: experience in 385 male patients. Chest 1988;94:9–14.

[19] Schwartz AR, Eisele DW, Smith PL. Pharyngeal airway obstruction in obstructive sleep apnea: pathophysiology and clinical implications. Otolaryngol Clin North Am 1998;31:911–8.

[20] Garrigue S, Bordier P, Jais P, et al. Benefit of atrial pacing in sleep apnea syndrome. N Engl J Med 2002;346:404–12.

[21] Roche F, Xuong AN, Court-Fortune I, et al. Relationship among the severity of sleep apnea syndrome, cardiac arrhythmias, and autonomic imbalance. Pacing Clin Electrophysiol 2003;26:669–77.

[22] Woodson BT, Brusky LT, Saurajen A, et al. Association of autonomic dysfunction and mild obstructive sleep apnea. Otolaryngol Head Neck Surg 2004;130:643–8.

[23] Zoccali C, Mallamaci F, Tripepi G, et al. Autonomic neuropathy is linked to nocturnal hypoxaemia and to concentric hypertrophy and remodelling in dialysis patients. Nephrol Dial Transplant 2001;16:70–7.

[24] Yun AJ, Lee PY, Bazar KA. Autonomic dysregulation as a basis of cardiovascular, endocrine, and inflammatory disturbances associated with obstructive sleep apnea and other conditions of chronic hypoxia, hypercapnia, and acidosis. Med Hypotheses 2004;62:852–6.

[25] Liu PY, Yee B, Wishart SM, et al. The short-term effects of high-dose testosterone on sleep, breathing, and function in older men. J Clin Endocrinol Metab 2003;88:3605–13.

[26] Stewart DA, Grunstein RR, Berthon-Jones M, et al. Androgen blockade does not affect sleep-disordered breathing or chemosensitivity in men with obstructive sleep apnea. Am Rev Respir Dis 1992;146:1389–93.

[27] Cunningham GR, Hirshkowitz M. Inhibition of steroid 5 alpha-reductase with finasteride: sleep-related erections, potency, and libido in healthy men. J Clin Endocrinol Metab 1995;80:1934–40.

[28] Bixler EO, Vgontzas AN, Lin HM, et al. Prevalence of sleep-disordered breathing in women: effects of gender. Am J Respir Crit Care Med 2001;163:608–13.

[29] Shahar E, Redline S, Young T, et al. Hormone replacement therapy and sleep-disordered breathing. Am J Respir Crit Care Med 2003;167:1186–92.

[30] Young T, Finn L, Austin D, et al. Menopausal status and sleep-disordered breathing in the Wisconsin Sleep Cohort Study. Am J Respir Crit Care Med 2003;167:1181–5.

[31] Rosenow F, McCarthy V, Caruso AC. Sleep apnoea in endocrine diseases. J Sleep Res 1998;7:3–11.

[32] Hochban W, Ehlenz K, Conradt R, et al. Obstructive sleep apnoea in acromegaly: the role of craniofacial changes. Eur Respir J 1999;14:196–202.

[33] Horner RL, Mohiaddin RH, Lowell DG, et al. Sites and sizes of fat deposits around the pharynx in obese patients with obstructive sleep apnoea and weight matched controls. Eur Respir J 1989;2:613–22.

[34] Bottini P, Dottorini ML, Cristina Cordoni M, et al. Sleep-disordered breathing in nonobese diabetic subjects with autonomic neuropathy. Eur Respir J 2003;22:654–60.

[35] Jokic R, Klimaszewski A, Mink J, et al. Surface tension forces in sleep apnea: the role of a soft tissue lubricant: a randomized double-blind, placebo-controlled trial. Am J Respir Crit Care Med 1998;157:1522–5.

[36] Kirkness JP, Madronio M, Stavrinou R, et al. Relationship between surface tension of upper airway lining liquid and upper airway collapsibility during sleep in obstructive sleep apnea hypopnea syndrome. J Appl Physiol 2003;95:1761–6.

[37] Schwartz AR, Schneider H, Smith PL. Upper airway surface tension: is it a significant cause of airflow obstruction during sleep? J Appl Physiol 2003;95:1759–60.

[38] Schlosshan D, Elliott MW. Sleep 3: clinical presentation and diagnosis of the obstructive sleep apnoea hypopnoea syndrome. Thorax 2004;59:347–52.

[39] Viner S, Szalai JP, Hoffstein V. Are history and physical examination a good screening test for sleep apnea? Ann Intern Med 1991;115:356–9.

[40] Partinen M, Guilleminault C. Daytime sleepiness and vascular morbidity at seven-year follow-up in obstructive sleep apnea patients. Chest 1990;97:27–32.

[41] Teran-Santos J, Jimenez-Gomez A, Cordero-Guevara J for the Cooperative Group Burgos-Santander. The association between sleep apnea and the risk of traffic accidents. N Engl J Med 1999;340:847–51.

[42] Powell NB, Schechtman KB, Riley RW, et al. Sleepy driving: accidents and injury. Otolaryngol Head Neck Surg 2002;126:217–27.

[43] Chervin RD, Zallek SN, Lin X, et al. Sleep disordered breathing in patients with cluster headache. Neurology 2000;54:2302–6.

[44] Richert A, Ansarin K, Baran AS. Sleep apnea and hypertension: pathophysiologic mechanisms. Semin Nephrol 2002;22:71–7.

[45] Bixler EO, Vgontzas AN, Lin HM, et al. Association of hypertension and sleep-disordered breathing. Arch Intern Med 2000;160:2289–95.

[46] Peppard PE, Young T, Palta M, et al. Prospective study of the association between sleep-disordered breathing and hypertension. N Engl J Med 2000;342:1378–84.

[47] Fletcher EC, Orolinova N, Bader M. Blood pressure response to chronic episodic hypoxia: the renin-angiotensin system. J Appl Physiol 2002;92:627–33.

[48] Moller DS, Lind P, Strunge B, et al. Abnormal vasoactive hormones and 24-hour blood pressure in obstructive sleep apnea. Am J Hypertens 2003;16:274–80.

[49] Ip MS, Lam B, Chan LY, et al. Circulating nitric oxide is suppressed in obstructive sleep apnea and is reversed by nasal continuous positive airway pressure. Am J Respir Crit Care Med 2000; 162:2166–71.

[50] Meslier N, Gagnadoux F, Giraud P, et al. Impaired glucose-insulin metabolism in males with obstructive sleep apnoea syndrome. Eur Respir J 2003;22:156–60.

[51] Vgontzas AN, Legro RS, Bixler EO, et al. Polycystic ovary syndrome is associated with obstructive sleep apnea and daytime sleepiness: role of insulin resistance. J Clin Endocrinol Metab 2001;86:517–20.

[52] Harsch IA, Schahin SP, Radespiel-Troger M, et al. Continuous positive airway pressure treatment rapidly improves insulin sensitivity in patients with obstructive sleep apnea syndrome. Am J Respir Crit Care Med 2004;169:156–62.

[53] Harsch IA, Schahin SP, Bruckner K, et al. The effect of continuous positive airway pressure treatment on insulin sensitivity in patients with obstructive sleep apnoea syndrome and type 2 diabetes. Respiration 2004;71:252–9.

[54] Punjabi NM, Ahmed MM, Polotsky VY, et al. Sleep-disordered breathing, glucose intolerance, and insulin resistance. Respir Physiol Neurobiol 2003;136:167–78.

[55] Stoohs RA, Facchini F, Guilleminault C. Insulin resistance and sleep-disordered breathing in healthy humans. Am J Respir Crit Care Med 1996;154:170–4.

[56] Shamsuzzaman AS, Somers VK. Fibrinogen, stroke, and obstructive sleep apnea: an evolving paradigm of cardiovascular risk. Am J Respir Crit Care Med 2000;162:2018–20.

[57] Franklin KA. Cerebral haemodynamics in obstructive sleep apnoea and Cheyne-Stokes respiration. Sleep Med Rev 2002;6:429–41.

[58] Szucs A, Vitrai J, Janszky J, et al. Pathological sleep apnea frequency remains permanent in ischaemic stroke and it is transient in haemorrhagic stroke. Eur Neurol 2002;47:15–9.

[59] Leung RS, Bradley TD. Sleep apnea and cardiovascular disease. Am J Respir Crit Care Med 2001;164:2147–65.

[60] Lanfranchi P, Somers VK. Obstructive sleep apnea and vascular disease. Respir Res 2001;2: 315–9.

[61] Nieto FJ, Herrington DM, Redline S, et al. Sleep apnea and markers of vascular endothelial function in a large community sample of older adults. Am J Respir Crit Care Med 2004;169: 354–60.

[62] Duchna HW, Guilleminault C, Stoohs RA, et al. Vascular reactivity in obstructive sleep apnea syndrome. Am J Respir Crit Care Med 2000;161:187–91.

[63] Grote L, Kraiczi H, Hedner J. Reduced alpha- and beta(2)-adrenergic vascular response in patients with obstructive sleep apnea. Am J Respir Crit Care Med 2000;162:1480–7.

[64] Dyugovskaya L, Lavie P, Lavie L. Increased adhesion molecules expression and production of reactive oxygen species in leukocytes of sleep apnea patients. Am J Respir Crit Care Med 2002;165:934–9.

[65] Bokinsky G, Miller M, Ault K, et al. Spontaneous platelet activation and aggregation during obstructive sleep apnea and its response to therapy with nasal continuous positive airway pressure: a preliminary investigation. Chest 1995;108:625–30.

[66] Mooe T, Franklin KA, Wiklund U, et al. Sleep-disordered breathing and myocardial ischemia in patients with coronary artery disease. Chest 2000;117:1597–602.

[67] Cherniack NS. Apnea and periodic breathing during sleep. N Engl J Med 1999;341:985–7.

[68] Chan J, Sanderson J, Chan W, et al. Prevalence of sleep-disordered breathing in diastolic heart failure. Chest 1997;111:1488–93.

[69] Guidry UC, Mendes LA, Evans JC, et al. Echocardiographic features of the right heart in sleep-disordered breathing: the Framingham Heart Study. Am J Respir Crit Care Med 2001;164: 933–8.

[70] Harbison J, O'Reilly P, McNicholas WT. Cardiac rhythm disturbances in the obstructive sleep apnea syndrome: effects of nasal continuous positive airway pressure therapy. Chest 2000;118: 591–5.

[71] Fichter J, Bauer D, Arampatzis S, et al. Sleep-related breathing disorders are associated with ventricular arrhythmias in patients with an implantable cardioverter-defibrillator. Chest 2002; 122:558–61.

[72] Samelson CF. Gastroesophageal reflux and obstructive sleep apnea. Sleep 1989;12:475–6.

[73] Graf KI, Karaus M, Heinemann S, et al. Gastroesophageal reflux in patients with sleep apnea syndrome. Z Gastroenterol 1995;33:689–93.

[74] Ing AJ, Ngu MC, Breslin AB. Obstructive sleep apnea and gastroesophageal reflux. Am J Med 2000;108(Suppl 4a):S120–2125.

[75] Green BT, Broughton WA, O'Connor JB. Marked improvement in nocturnal gastroesophageal reflux in a large cohort of patients with obstructive sleep apnea treated with continuous positive airway pressure. Arch Intern Med 2003;163:41–5.

[76] Steward DL. Pantoprazole for sleepiness associated with acid reflux and obstructive sleep disordered breathing. Laryngoscope 2004;114:1525–8.

[77] Valipour A, Makker HK, Hardy R, et al. Symptomatic gastroesophageal reflux in subjects with a breathing sleep disorder. Chest 2002;121:1748–53.

[78] Ozturk O, Ozturk L, Ozdogan A, et al. Variables affecting the occurrence of gastroesophageal reflux in obstructive sleep apnea patients. Eur Arch Otorhinolaryngol 2004;261:229–32.

ELSEVIER
SAUNDERS

Anesthesiology Clin N Am
23 (2005) 445–461

ANESTHESIOLOGY
CLINICS OF
NORTH AMERICA

The Biology and Genetics of Obesity and Obstructive Sleep Apnea

Avery Tung, MD

Department of Anesthesia and Critical Care, University of Chicago, 5841 South Maryland Avenue,
MC4028, Chicago, IL 60637, USA

Although richly detailed clinical descriptions of the obstructive sleep apnea (OSA) syndrome have existed since the 19th Century [1], our understanding of the origins, causes, and risk factors underlying OSA remains incompletely understood today. At first glance, the influence of genetics on the pathogenesis of sleep apnea appears relatively straightforward. All patients with OSA exhibit repetitive obstruction of the upper airway during sleep, episodic arterial oxygen desaturation, spontaneous arousals, sleep fragmentation, and daytime hypersomnolence [2]. The severity of sleep apnea is assessed using the apnea-hypopnea index (AHI), defined as the number of episodes of breathing obstruction that exceeds a certain duration (usually ≥ 10 s/hour of sleep) [3]. Given this definition, it seems reasonable that associated factors such as obesity would predispose patients to OSA by narrowing the upper airway and increasing the likelihood of airway obstruction. If this logic is taken further, it is also reasonable to imagine that genetically mediated malformations of the upper airway or a genetic predisposition to obesity would thus facilitate the expression of OSA.

Although it seems straightforward, proving this line of reasoning is complicated by several issues. All patients with sleep apnea exhibit repetitive, episodic airway obstruction, and the most common risk factors for the syndrome include male gender, an age of 40 or more years old, and obesity. Not all patients present with these characteristics, however [4]. Attempts to construct causal relationships between potential genetic risk factors and the clinical presentation of OSA must therefore account for this variability in presentation. In addition, it is unclear whether factors associated with sleep apnea are causes or effects of the syndrome. Although it is reasonable to consider obesity an associated condi-

E-mail address: atung@dacc.uchicago.edu

tion that increases the risk for sleep apnea, for example, it may also be that the daytime hypersomnolence typical of sleep apnea predisposes to obesity by decreasing daytime activity. Such difficulty in determining the causal direction of these associations increases the challenge of identifying and understanding how risk factors for OSA relate to the disease. Finally, because little is known about brain function during sleep, the relative contributions of ventilatory control abnormalities and sleep regulatory abnormalities, obesity, and sleep deprivation to apneic episodes during sleep remain a mystery.

Although many attempts to understand and treat sleep apnea have revolved around environmental factors such as weight loss and anatomical reconstruction of abnormal airways, recent evidence suggests that genetic variability may play a significant causal role in the pathogenesis of OSA. Multiple studies [5] of the prevalence of sleep apnea among relatives of affected patients indicate that a positive family history of OSA is an important risk factor for an elevated AHI and consequences such as snoring and daytime sleepiness. Moreover, clear familial linkages have been described for several "intermediate" phenotypes likely to contribute to the sleep apnea syndrome. Segregation analysis, for example, has suggested that up to 40% of the variation in body mass index (BMI) and fat mass may be the result of a genetic variation between different ethnic groups [6] and that altered ventilatory responses to hypoxemia and or hypercapnia also may be partly attributable to genetic factors [7]. This article reviews the current knowledge about a genetic approach to the causes and risk factors for sleep apnea, examines the data supporting a genetic influence on sleep apnea, and discusses how the presence of such factors might play a clinical role in the perioperative management of patients with sleep apnea.

Definitions, thresholds, and methodology

Because of complexities in describing and quantifying sleep apnea, significant difficulties arise in determining to what degree sleep apnea is a genetic phenomenon. Although much of the literature focuses on the AHI as both a definition of sleep apnea and a measure of its severity, this measure is limited in two important ways. First, although an apnea is relatively easy to define (cessation of airflow for ≥ 10 s), no consensus agreement exists for a definition of hypopnea [8]. Because hypopnea occurs approximately twice as often as apnea [9], this lack of agreement can affect the variability of an AHI measurement. In 2001, the American Academy of Sleep Medicine [10] defined a hypopneic episode as an abnormal respiratory event lasting at least 10 seconds, with a reduction of at least 30% in thoracoabdominal movement or airflow relative to baseline and an oxygen desaturation of at least 4%. Despite this definition, many laboratories continue to use different approaches [11].

In addition, although detecting an apneic episode is relatively simple, detecting a hypopneic episode requires a quantitative assessment of airflow or of body movement. Because measuring airflow directly requires the use of a close fitting mask, it is technically impractical during most clinical sleep studies. As a result, routine evaluation of airflow during a sleep study is usually made by measuring changes in the temperature or CO_2 content of inspired versus expired gases [11]. Assessments of thoracoabdominal motion are also made indirectly, leading to large potential sources of variation. It is easy to see how differences in the definition of hypopnea can lead to variability in the diagnosis of sleep apnea and thus the difficulty of determining the relative contribution of genetic factors.

Finally, although threshold values of the AHI ($\cong 15$) correlate with the risk of hypertension and cardiovascular morbidity [12], the AHI alone does not adequately assess the impact of sleep apnea on daytime behavior or on quality of life. Patients with mild sleep apnea, for example (AHI $\cong 5$), may or may not have life-altering symptoms of sleep apnea (daytime sleepiness, impaired cognition, or mood disorders) [13]. Such symptoms may be more (or less) heritable than are indicated by the AHI and thus may be overvalued or undervalued when using the AHI alone to determine genetic origins. In addition, because snoring is relatively frequent [14], a higher threshold value for the AHI would likely result in a reduced estimate of genetic contribution.

Although the AHI is not uniformly defined and is difficult to measure and requires a threshold for significance, it remains the most commonly used tool to diagnose and assess the magnitude of sleep apnea [3]. As a result, most of the data supporting a genetic role in the pathogenesis of sleep apnea are derived from studies that use the AHI (at varying thresholds) as their primary diagnostic tool. For anesthesiologists, it is thus reasonable to imagine that higher AHI values indicate a greater severity of disease and more severe sleep fragmentation. In light of animal data suggesting a potentiating effect of sleep deprivation on anesthetic potency [15], patients with more severe OSA may be more sensitive to anesthetic agents.

Familial relationships in sleep apnea

Most physicians are familiar with the prototypical presentation of sleep apnea, including obesity, hypertension, daytime hypersomnolence, and a history of snoring. Not all patients with sleep apnea, however, have such clearly visible symptoms. A growing recognition of the importance of sleep apnea in the perioperative (and particularly the postoperative) period suggests that increasing the sensitivity of diagnosis during preoperative evaluation may potentially alter anesthetic management. One such screening measure is the presence or absence of family members with sleep apnea.

Does a history of OSA in first-degree relatives increase a patient's risk of having OSA? Both case reports and several large studies suggest this possibility. One early report of a possible familial element to the genesis of sleep apnea was published in 1978 [16]. In a family with five sons, four of five sons had been diagnosed with sleep apnea, one had died while asleep, and one son's child died from sudden infant death syndrome. The authors suggest a "genetic abnormality of respiratory muscle control," and noted that family members of patients diagnosed with sleep apnea may be at higher risk for the syndrome. Although other case reports with similar anecdotal findings were subsequently reported [17], the first large scale systematic efforts did not appear until the 1990s. One 1992 study [5] used questionnaires to compare the sleep habits of 163 relatives of 29 patients with sleep apnea with those of 109 control subjects. The authors found that the odds ratio (OR) of having "breathing pauses" was significantly elevated for relatives of patients with sleep apnea, ranging from 1.4 with one affected relative to 3.1 with three relatives. Similar ratios were observed in that study for snoring and daytime sleepiness. That these ratios persisted after adjustment for age, gender, and body mass index lent further support to a hypothesized genetic component to sleep apnea.

A subsequent study [18] by the same authors used home or laboratory monitoring to verify the diagnosis of sleep apnea in first-degree relatives and also found a relationship between sleep apnea and familial factors. Using a threshold AHI of 15, the odds ratio of having sleep apnea was 1.6 with one affected relative and 3.9 with three relatives. These data were significant even after adjustment for age, gender, race, and body mass index. Another polysomnographic comparison between relatives of patients with sleep apnea and control subjects demonstrated a higher incidence of sleep apneas (13 versus 4/h, respectively), more arousals (30 versus 17/h, respectively), and more oxygen desaturation in relatives [19]. In that study, the authors also observed longer soft palates, wider uvulae, and narrower upper airways and postulated that the familial component may result partly from differences in facial structure.

Although these studies were unable to identify specific genetic elements that may have contributed to a familial link in the genesis of sleep apnea, they did suggest potential clues. First, despite the likelihood that obesity is partly genetically mediated and that it predisposes to sleep apnea, the above studies all found evidence for a genetic link independent of BMI. Subsequently, more specific genomic analyses [20] have supported significant linkages for the AHI, even when adjusted for BMI and vice versa. Second, symptoms such as snoring also appear to have a familial transmission pattern. In addition to the studies noted above, other investigators have observed a significant concordance for snoring among twins and that a family history of snoring represents a risk factor, with the odds ratio for snoring ranging from 2.5 to 4.2 depending on the type of family relationship (grandparent versus parent) [21]. Although snoring may be partly related to upper airway fat deposition, these data retain significance after adjustments for obesity (BMI) and suggest an actual disorder of breathing muscle regulation. It is known, for example, that to prevent airway collapse, upper airway muscles activate approximately 100 ms before inspiratory muscle activity during sleep in normal subjects [22]. This activation occurs to a lesser degree or not at all, however, in patients with sleep apnea [23]. The genesis for this abnormality is unclear and may relate to as yet poorly understood genetic factors.

For anesthesiologists, these data suggest that asking about family history during the preoperative evaluation may significantly increase the sensitivity of screening for sleep apnea. Although obesity, hypertension, and snoring are more visible clues to the diagnosis, family members with sleep apnea appear to confer the same degree of risk and may represent a different causal mechanism with potentially greater anesthetic consequences.

Specific genes and genetic markers associated with sleep apnea

In addition to family studies, researchers have also attempted to understand the genetic contribution to sleep apnea by mapping the genome of high-risk populations. The colocalization of specific genetic regions and gene markers with sleep apnea is in part hampered by the complexity of the syndrome and variability in the diagnosis. Nevertheless, associations between sleep apnea and known genetic markers have been observed. In white subjects, whole-genome scans implicate regions on chromosomes 1p, 2p, 12p, and 19p with sleep apnea, and in African Americans, chromosome 8q appears to be a possible candidate [20]. Certain genetic markers also correlate with sleep apnea. A 1993 study of Japanese patients with sleep apnea observed an increased incidence of the HLA-A2 and -B39 antigens [24]. When snoring was used as a surrogate for sleep apnea, a higher incidence of the Lewis blood group phenotype Le(a+b+) was noted [21]. Because of a higher incidence of hypertension and diabetes in patients with sleep apnea, associations between genes controlling expression of angiotensin-converting enzyme (ACE) inhibitors and sleep apnea have been examined. Although some preliminary results have suggested a relationship [25], other studies [26] suggest that the effects of polymorphisms in genes controlling ACE expression may be confounded by hypertension. Finally, a high incidence of apnea in patients with Alzheimer's disease has raised the possibility that genetic markers for Alzheimer's disease such as apolipoprotein E ε4 (APOEε4) may also associate with sleep apnea [27]. Although one large study of 791 patients observed a higher likelihood of sleep apnea in patients with APOEε4 [28], the differences were not large and were not replicated in another, similar study [29].

Currently, the anesthetic relevance of specific genetic markers is unclear. Because sleep apnea is a complex syndrome with multiple causative factors, even a complete understanding of the genetic predisposition may not predict the clinical presentation. As a result, the use of genetic markers for preoperative predictive purposes is not likely to be any better than the combination of clinical criteria and patient history. Although in the future an understanding of the precise genetic contribution to sleep apnea may allow meaningful therapy, the role of specific genes or gene markers in sleep apnea is currently limited.

Obesity and sleep apnea

If genetic factors play a role in the pathogenesis of sleep apnea, how might those factors manifest? Although it is possible that genetic factors operate completely independently from known risk factors for sleep apnea, it may also be that genetic factors enhance the heritability of "intermediate" phenotypes with clear relationships to sleep apnea. Obesity is perhaps the best example of this type of trait. It is likely that obesity is partly genetically mediated and almost certain that obesity contributes to the onset of sleep apnea. Although not all patients with sleep apnea are overweight, obesity (defined by a BMI ≥ 28) remains, along with male gender, one of the most characteristic features of sleep apnea [30]. Epidemiologic studies indicate that obesity is present in 60% to 90% of patients evaluated in sleep clinics [4]. Moreover, increases in the degree of obesity correlate to increases in the severity and prevalence of sleep apnea. In a 1993 study [31] of 602 subjects prescreened for sleep disorders and habitual snoring, each increase of 10 kg in body weight doubled the odds ratio for sleep-disordered breathing. Supporting a genetic element in the relationship between obesity and sleep apnea was the added significance of where the fat was distributed. The OR for sleep-disordered breathing was even higher (OR, 3.4) for each 0.09 increase in waist-hip ratio and higher yet (OR, 5) for each 4.5-cm increase in neck girth. Other studies [32] have observed that patients with severe sleep apnea (AHI ~ 40) have larger lateral pharyngeal wall volumes, tongues, and upper airway soft tissue than control subjects and that each 3-mm increase in pharyngeal fat thickness resulted in a 6-fold increase in the likelihood for sleep apnea.

The above data demonstrate that the distribution of fat may be an even more significant factor than overall weight for the genesis of sleep apnea. Fat localized on the upper body or on the neck and parapharyngeal area indicates a significantly higher risk for sleep apnea than fat alone.

Existing evidence strongly suggests that different patterns of regional fat deposition in obese patients represent entirely different syndromes [33]. At a cellular level, upper body abdominal and visceral fat is more metabolically active and has a greater β-adrenergic lipolytic sensitivity than femoral and gluteal fat in the "pear"-shaped body. Lower body fat, most common in women, is metabolically less active and available [33]. These different obese phenotypes not only have different cellular characteristics but also produce dramatically different metabolic consequences at the systemic level. Rates of insulin resistance, hypertension, diabetes, unfavorable lipid profiles, stroke, and coronary artery disease are all higher with upper body fat patterns than with lower, indicating that upper body, "apple"-shaped fat patterns are fundamentally different from lower body, pear-shaped distributions.

Such phenotypic differences support a role for genetics in obesity. Measures of fat deposition such as the waist-hip ratio suggest that 30% to 35% of the variance in obesity pattern can be accounted for by a multifactorial inheritance pattern or a major gene locus [34]. Twin studies of overfeeding also support an element of genetic control over fat distribution. In nearly all such studies, variability in weight gain with overfeeding was greater among twin pairs than within pairs; for example, a 1990 study of 12 pairs of adult male identical twins found more than six times as much variance among than within pairs with respect to abdominal visceral fat and regional fat distribution [35].

For anesthesiologists, the implications of the relationship between obesity, fat distribution, and sleep apnea are fairly straightforward. First, BMI alone may not be as effective a screening tool for sleep apnea as measurements of regional fat distribution such as neck circumference. Second, fat associated with metabolic and cardiovascular consequences may be more predictive of sleep apnea than fat in the absence of those consequences. Finally, these data underscore the concept that, although it is underdiagnosed, sleep apnea is a complex syndrome with a wide variety of associated factors and that ruling out the diagnosis on the basis of a single measurement such as BMI may be problematic.

Mechanisms linking genetic variability in obesity and sleep apnea

What mechanisms might link genetic differences among individuals, differences in the propensity toward obesity, and sleep apnea? Polygenic studies have identified only weak associations between obesity and numerous genes involved in energy expenditure. Polymorphisms in mitochondrial uncoupling proteins, β_2 and β_3 adrenoceptors (which have antiobesity effects in animals), and peroxisome proliferator-activated receptors, which stimulate adipocyte growth, have only been weakly associated with obesity [36]. Mendelian syndromes involving obesity, such as Prader-Willi syndrome or Albright's hereditary osteodystrophy, can be traced to specific genes on specific chromosomes and are another possible model for genetic effects on obesity. These syndromes, however, are associated with other significantly abnormal characteristics and clearly do not represent the majority of obese patients.

Single gene mutations in hormone-receptor systems that result in obesity alone have been described in individual case reports. Mutations in the genes for proopiomelanocortin, the melanocortin-4 receptor, and carboxypeptidases responsible for post-translational conversion of neuroendocrine pro-hormones have all been associated with an adiposity that is frequently severe [37]. Although our understanding of these genotype-phenotype relationships is now slightly better, they are also unlikely to explain more than a small fraction of obese subjects.

With respect to sleep apnea, one potentially important factor linking genetic variation to obesity is leptin. A polypeptide hormone secreted by adipocytes, leptin circulates at levels proportional to body fat content and penetrates into the cerebrospinal fluid (CSF) to act on leptin receptors in the hypothalamus [38]. In normal human metabolism, low leptin levels act to trigger a complex series of neuroendocrine responses that increase energy intake and decrease energy consumption. Subjects homozygous for a mutation resulting in an abnormal leptin structure exhibit not only severe hyperphagia and extreme obesity [39] but also a resolution of their condition with exogenous leptin administration [40]. Interestingly, heterozygous relatives of these subjects also were found to have lower leptin levels and obesity.

In most obese patients, however, leptin levels are elevated and not depressed [41]. Moreover, when obese patients with high leptin levels lose weight, their leptin levels decrease accordingly [42]. These seemingly discordant observations may be explained by the observation that the ratio of CSF to serum leptin levels decreases with BMI [43]. As a result, although more leptin is circulating in the serum, less of it may potentially be acting at relevant hypothalamic receptors. Taken together, these observations suggest that predominant features of most obese humans are an elevated leptin level and what may be best described as a syndrome of leptin resistance [44].

Evidence exists to suggest that leptin levels may be one factor linking genetic influences to phenotypes at high risk for sleep apnea. Leptin levels appear to be at least partly genetically governed [45] and may correlate with fat distribution as well as BMI. In addition, studies [46] in patients with sleep apnea demonstrate that regions of chromosomes 2p, 3p, 4p, and 21p are significantly linked to plasma leptin levels. When corrected for BMI, women have much lower leptin levels than men, mirroring the lower incidence of sleep apnea in women [47]. Serum leptin levels are also elevated in patients with sleep apnea and appear to correlate strongly with the apnea-hypopnea index [48]. That this correlation is diminished after adjustment for obesity suggests that the correlation between leptin and AHI results from leptin effects on energy balance and obesity [48]. Finally, the high leptin levels associated with sleep apnea decrease when nasal continuous positive airway pressure therapy (CPAP) is applied [49]. Although it is unclear how CPAP reduces leptin levels, this finding further supports a hypothesis that elevated leptin levels are involved in the pathogenesis of sleep apnea.

In addition to its effects on obesity, leptin may also play a role in the regulation of breathing. Both hypercapnia and hypoxia appear to increase leptin levels in animal models. Studies [50] in leptin-deficient mice demonstrate not only obesity but also a rapid breathing pattern and a blunted response to hypercapnia compared with normal subjects. This reduced responsiveness to CO_2 was present before the onset of obesity, and when combined with a rapid breathing pattern resulted in an elevated resting partial (P)CO_2 level. Interestingly, the decreased responsiveness to hypercapnia in leptin-deficient mice was particularly marked during sleep, with nearly no response to hypercapnia during rapid eye movement (REM) sleep [50]. In these mice, 3 days of leptin replacement therapy (administered acutely to avoid confounding effects of changes in weight) normalized CO_2 responsiveness during both non-(N)REM and REM sleep but not during wakefulness [51].

Leptin may also have a role in the regulation of sleep. Leptin receptors are present in the dorsal raphe and the reticular activating system, nuclei known to be involved in arousal [52]. Both levels of leptin and the leptin receptor fluctuate with time of day, suggesting a circadian influence on leptin signaling [53]. In addition, the administration of orexins A and B, polypeptides known to regulate sleep state, appears to increase leptin levels [54]. Finally, in animals, leptin appears to increase NREM sleep and decrease REM sleep as long as caloric intake is maintained [55]. Behaviorally, changes in sleep also modulate leptin levels. In healthy, nonobese patients who were subjected to 2 days of chronic sleep deprivation (≤ 4 hours per night), leptin levels were reduced by 18% [56]. This finding suggests that sleep deprivation is partly perceived by the body as a state of energy deficit. Although the effects of sleep deprivation on leptin levels seem to conflict with the high leptin levels commonly seen in sleep apnea, it may be that chronic oxygen desaturation and hypercapnia, stimuli known to increase leptin levels, are more important than sleep deprivation. It may also be that responses to sleep deprivation in healthy nonobese subjects differ from those in obese patients with sleep apnea. In any case, elevated leptin levels in OSA may be more than a metabolic consequence of the syndrome.

Taken together, the potential links between sleep homeostasis, leptin levels, obesity, and control of breathing suggest a route by which genetic influences can allow sleep apnea to manifest under the right environmental conditions. Because the full role of leptin in normal and obese physiology has yet to be elucidated, it is difficult to integrate the role of leptin into the pathogenesis of sleep apnea. Nevertheless, we know that sleep deprivation induces low leptin levels and increased appetite in normal subjects. It is also clear that obesity is a leptin-resistant state in which leptin levels are high and that this resistance may occur because of impaired leptin transport from the blood to the CSF. Low leptin levels blunt the respiratory response to hypercapnia, and leptin appears to be a respiratory stimulant. Both episodic hypoxia and hypercapnia increase leptin levels. Finally, leptin alters sleep patterns.

Because leptin physiology is so unclear, the anesthetic implications of understanding the link between leptin and sleep apnea are unclear. It appears that general anesthesia lowers leptin levels [57] but that postoperatively leptin levels return to normal [58]. The relevance of such a perioperative change in leptin levels remains unknown. Presently, no evidence exists to support the use of leptin either as a screening or therapeutic tool in the perioperative management of patients.

Other inherited phenotypes that predispose to sleep apnea

Craniofacial morphology

Another reasonable mechanism by which human genetic variability might predispose to sleep apnea is through structural abnormalities of the bony and soft tissues that reduce the size of the upper airway. A number of characteristic craniofacial differences have been observed when patients with sleep apnea are compared with age-matched and gender-matched controls. Specifically, patients with sleep apnea tend to have a retroposed maxilla and mandible, a narrow posterior airway, an enlarged tongue and soft palate, and an inferiorly positioned hyoid bone [59]. An increased likelihood of enlarged parapharyngeal fat pads has also been described in patients with sleep apnea [32]. Taken together, these changes have a common effect of narrowing the upper airway.

Evidence suggests that the presence of specific craniofacial abnormalities that narrow the airway during wakefulness translates into an increased risk for sleep apnea. In one CT study [60] of upper airway size, for example, reduced upper airway patency correlated with both the rate of sleep-disordered breathing and the degree of oxygen desaturation. Another radiographic study [61] of 155 patients with sleep apnea (respiratory disturbance index ≥ 10) observed craniofacial dimensions that were significantly different (≥ 2 standard deviations) than a control group of 41 normal patients. Both the extent and specificity of the craniofacial abnormalities observed were notable. Only two of 155 patients had normal dimensions, and common findings included a normal maxilla, retroposed mandible, more acute angle of flexure of the cranial base, and an inferior displacement of the hyoid bone. As expected, the combined sum of these changes increased the length of the soft palate and reduced the space occupied by airway soft tissues. Specific cephalometric models targeting abnormalities characteristic of sleep apnea have also successfully identified patients with sleep apnea, when used prospectively. One model, combining measures of obesity (neck circumference and BMI) with cephalomorphic data (mandibular width and length), demonstrated 97.6% sensitivity and 100% specificity for the diagnosis of sleep apnea, when applied to patients evaluated for sleep disorders [62].

As expected, several lines of evidence support the presence of a genetic influence on craniofacial abnormalities that correlate with sleep apnea. Pediatric syndromes with associated craniofacial abnormalities, such as Treacher Collins or Pierre Robin syndrome, involve mandibular hypoplasia and appear to be at least partly caused by genetic influences. In addition, the relationship between craniofacial abnormalities and sleep apnea appears to differ among different races. In whites, for example, a cephalic index (ratio of head width to anteroposterior head length) greater than 0.8 represents an increased risk for sleep apnea [63]. In contrast, no increase in risk is seen in African Americans with this head shape [64]. It is unclear whether this relationship holds in Asians, who have a higher prevalence of the brachycephalic head shape in which craniofacial indices exceed 0.8. Observations that both soft tissue and bony abnormalities correlate with sleep apnea in whites, whereas only soft tissue differences appear to be relevant to African Americans [64], further identify race as a potentially important variable in the relationships among craniofacial morphology, genetics, and sleep apnea.

Craniofacial changes associated with sleep apnea also appear to have a familial and thus a potentially genetic basis. Twin studies [65,66] indicate high heritability estimates for a number of craniofacial features that correlate with OSA. Among these features is the cephalic index, which carries an estimated heritability of 0.9 in males and 0.7 in females [65]. When dental malocclusions are studied, a significant contribution of heredity is also seen [66].

Although craniofacial abnormalities themselves do not explain the sleep-induced dysregulation of ventilatory control that characterizes sleep apnea, they correlate with both inheritance patterns and sleep apnea sufficiently strongly enough to suggest a significant contribution. From an anesthetic point of view, these correlations appear sufficiently strong enough to indicate they may have a role in preoperative screening, particularly when the baseline incidence of sleep apnea is high. When combined with estimates of adiposity (neck size and BMI), race, or a personal history suggestive of OSA, a craniofacial evaluation of the likelihood of sleep apnea may be of benefit in a sufficiently high-risk population.

Alterations in ventilatory control

Although anatomic abnormalities may predispose to sleep apnea, a defect in the neurologic control of breathing during sleep is also required for the syndrome to manifest. Studies of neural activity during sleep demonstrate two clear differences between patients with sleep apnea and those without. In normal subjects, upper airway activity begins before respiratory "pump" activity occurs, tensing the soft tissues to prevent them from collapsing during inspiratory airflow. In patients with sleep apnea, however, this synchronization of upper airway and respiratory muscle activation is disrupted [67]. The result is inspiratory airflow occurring in the presence of a collapsible upper airway and an apneic episode. Another difference is that in normal subjects, decreases in oxygen saturation result in a short-term potentiation of ventilatory effort. This potentiation facilitates ventilatory stability and decreases the likelihood of periodic or dysrhythmic breathing. In contrast, patients with sleep apnea demonstrate less potentiation, a prolonged desaturation resulting from apneic or hypopneic episodes, and periodic breathing [68]. Finally, patients with obstructive sleep apnea may also have central apneic episodes, suggesting fundamental abnormalities in the chemoreceptor or mechanoreceptor feedback loop governing normal ventilation [69].

Evidence exists to indicate that some aspect of these ventilatory abnormalities may be genetically mediated. A Japanese study [70] of 28 monozygotic and 10 dizygotic twins examined the ventilatory response to hypoxia, hypercapnia, and respiratory loading. Although the means were not different, the variance in both the hypoxic and hypercapnic drives were four to five times greater in dizygotic than in monozygotic twins. Another study [71] examined the ventilatory response to hypoxemia and hypercarbia in 14 adults with chronic obstructive pulmonary disease and 23 of their adult children. The authors found no relationship between hypercarbic drive and relatedness but did find an intergenerational correlation for hypoxic drive. Other, similar studies have also observed a high heritability for hypoxic drive in specific populations. A study [72] of Tibetans living at high altitude, for example, has suggested the presence of a major gene influencing 21% of the phenotypic variation in oxygen saturation. Overall, the data suggest that genetic variability plays a significant role both in the timing of airway muscle activity that occurs during sleep and in the ventilatory response to hypoxia.

Genetic effects on ventilatory control and function are likely to be relevant in sleep apnea. Children with congenital central hypoventilation syndromes not only have periodic apneas but also depressed hypercapnic and hypoxic ventilatory responses [73]. These syndromes have been correlated with mutations of several specific genes [74]. In adults with sleep apnea, familial studies also support a role for genetically based ventilatory control abnormalities in sleep apnea. In one such study [75], family members of patients with sleep apnea who also had sleep apnea were compared with relatives of patients without sleep apnea and with unrelated control subjects. Although responses to hypercapnia were similar among the groups, the response to hypoxia was blunted in family members both with and without sleep apnea relative to controls. Significant increases in airway resistance were also noted among family members with sleep apnea, suggesting that a combination of anatomical and ventilatory control factors is required for expression of the syndrome.

The perioperative relevance of ventilatory control abnormalities in patients with sleep apnea is unclear. Although the effects of inhaled anesthetics on normal control of respiration have been well studied, little is known about the effects of anesthetics on patients with abnormal respiratory drive. In normal humans, large variations in hypercapnic and hypoxic respiratory drive exist despite adjustment for age or sex [76]. In two strains of mice inbred for variable reductions in ventilatory responsiveness to CO_2, the administration of isoflurane anesthesia abolished interstrain differences [77]. During recovery, however, differences in the respiratory responsiveness to CO_2 reappeared and were magnified when compared with preoperative levels. In another, similar study [78], no differences were found among isoflurane, sevoflurane, and desflurane in their effect on CO_2 responsiveness. When these data are extrapolated to humans with sleep apnea, it would seem that intraoperative differences resulting from genetic influences on ventilatory control are minor. Ultimately, these data underscore the importance of the postoperative period in patients with sleep apnea.

Abnormalities in sleep regulation

Muscle tone is known to be reduced in non-rapid eye movement sleep and nearly absent in rapid eye movement sleep. Genetic variability in sleep regulation may therefore be another mechanism by which genes affect the expression of sleep apnea. Abnormalities in the stability of sleep and waking states or in the neuromuscular manifestation of state characteristics may all plausibly increase either the severity or frequency of apneic episodes. As the molecular basis for differences in sleep-state regulation becomes increasingly understood, recognizing abnormalities in sleep regulation may be another tool in diagnosing sleep apnea or predicting its perioperative consequences.

Narcolepsy is one disorder of sleep regulation that may play an important role in sleep apnea. Patients with narcolepsy characteristically suffer from hypersomnolence, disturbed nocturnal sleep, cataplexy, and sleep-onset REM periods [79]. In humans, a clear genetic component to narcolepsy is reflected in the observation that first-degree relatives of patients with narcolepsy have a risk of narcolepsy that is more than 10-fold higher than in normal subjects [80]. In dogs, deficits in the hypocretin receptor result in a canine form of narcolepsy, whereas in mice, gene-knockout models demonstrate that behavior similar to human narcolepsy results from deficiencies in orexin synthesis [80].

The orexin (also called hypocretin) system may represent another mechanism linking genetic variability and sleep apnea. Orexins are neuropeptides with behavioral effects on both the vigilance state and appetite control. Orexin-containing neurons, which are produced in the posterior hypothalamus, project widely to monoaminergic cell groups such as the locus coeruleus and tuberomamillary nucleus, as well as to other hypothalamic areas [80]. Two distinct receptors exist (orexin receptors 1 and 2) and have different distributions within the brain, suggesting different functional roles. Although the specific role for orexins in behavioral regulation is unclear, animal studies demonstrate that orexins stimulate both food intake and wakefulness. One hypothesis is that orexins are elaborated during fasting states to increase appetite and increase wakefulness to promote success in finding food.

In patients with sleep apnea, abnormalities in orexin regulation may also have a causative role. The affects of orexins on appetite control and arousal make them plausible candidates for a syndrome such as sleep apnea in which obesity is so prevalent. Preliminary data suggest that orexin levels are abnormal in patients with OSA. In one study [81], morning orexin levels were significantly lower in patients with sleep apnea than in controls. In a repeat study [82] examining orexin levels later in the day, this difference persisted. Another study [83] found low orexin levels in patients with sleep apnea but also found that reduced orexin levels with sleep apnea did not correlate either with BMI, treatment with CPAP, or with daytime hypersomnolence. These relationships suggest that orexin levels may not necessarily be a consequence of the syndrome but instead may be involved in the pathogenesis of sleep apnea. Because abnormalities in orexin synthesis or signaling may be genetically mediated, future work may reveal sleep state control as an important genetic factor in sleep apnea.

For anesthesiologists, too little is known about the relationships among narcolepsy, orexin, and sleep apnea to significantly change clinical practice. It is worth noting, however, that narcolepsy is also underdiagnosed, many narcoleptics are obese, the daytime hypersomnolence characteristic of the disease may theoretically lead to an increased sensitivity to anesthetics, and that many narcoleptics receive stimulant drugs that can interact with anesthesia and surgical stimulation.

Summary

Sleep apnea is a complex clinical syndrome with profound implications for perioperative care. Associations with hypertension, cardiovascular disease, and obesity make the intraoperative care of such patients extremely challenging, and an increased sensitivity to anesthetic agents dramatically increases the difficulty of postoperative care. Understanding the genetic bases for obesity and sleep apnea may have several long-term benefits for anesthesiologists. Because sleep apnea is chronically underdiagnosed, most patients with the disease will not carry a diagnosis at the time they present for anesthetic care. The inclusion of focused risk assessment tools and genetic markers in preoperative screening may increase the sensitivity of existing screening tests and reduce the number of patients who undergo anesthesia with undiagnosed sleep apnea. In addition, a greater insight into the relationship between genetic variance and sleep apnea may ultimately allow anesthesiologists to determine which patients with sleep apnea represent greater perioperative risks and thus which patients require special precautions. Finally, the increasing penetration of genetic knowledge into clinical medicine raises the future possibility that therapeutic options based on genetic diagnoses may allow anesthesiologists to modify either the expression of the disorder or its perioperative risk.

References

[1] Dickens C. The Pickwick papers. London: Penguin Books; 1999.
[2] Bassiri AG, Guilleminant C. Clinical features and evaluation of obstructive sleep apnea-hypopnea syndrome. In: Kryger MH, Roth T, Dement WC, editors. Principles and practice of sleep medicine. Philadelphia: WB Saunders; 2000. p. 869–78.
[3] van Houwelingen KG, van Uffelen R, van Vliet AC. The sleep apnoea syndromes. Eur Heart J 1999;20:858–66.
[4] Strohl KP, Redline S. Recognition of obstructive sleep apnea. Am J Respir Crit Care Med 1996; 154:279–89.
[5] Redline S, Tosteson T, Tishler PV, et al. Studies in the genetics of obstructive sleep apnea: familial aggregation of symptoms associated with sleep-related breathing disturbances. Am Rev Respir Dis 1992;145:440–4.
[6] Comuzzie AG, Allison DB. The search for human obesity genes. Science 1998;280:1374–7.
[7] el Bayadi S, Millman RP, Tishler PV, et al. A family study of sleep apnea: anatomic and physiologic interactions. Chest 1990;98:554–9.
[8] Redline S, Sanders M. Hypopnca, a floating metric: implications for prevalence, morbidity estimates, and case finding. Sleep 1997;20:1209–17.
[9] Block AJ, Boysen PG, Wynne JW, et al. Sleep apnea, hypopnea and oxygen desaturation in normal subjects: a strong male predominance. N Engl J Med 1979;300:513–7.
[10] Meoli AL, Casey KR, Clark RW, et al for the Clinical Practice Review Committee of the American Academy of Sleep Medicine. Hypopnea in sleep-disordered breathing in adults. Sleep 2001;24:469–70.
[11] Tsai WH, Flemons WW, Whitelaw WA, et al. A comparison of apnea-hypopnea indices derived from different definitions of hypopnea. Am J Respir Crit Care Med 1999;159:43–8.
[12] Carlson JT, Hedner JA, Ejnell H, et al. High prevalence of hypertension in sleep apnea patients independent of obesity. Am J Respir Crit Care Med 1994;150:72–7.
[13] Flemons WW, McNicholas WT. Clinical prediction of the sleep apnea syndrome. Sleep Med Rev 1997;1:19–32.
[14] Norton PG, Dunn EV, Haight JS. Snoring in adults: some epidemiologic aspects. Can Med Assoc J 1983;128:674–5.
[15] Tung A, Szafran MJ, Bluhm B, et al. Sleep deprivation potentiates the onset and duration of loss of righting reflex induced by propofol and isoflurane. Anesthesiology 2002;97:906–11.
[16] Strohl KP, Saunders NA, Feldman NT, et al. Obstructive sleep apnea in family members. N Engl J Med 1978;299:969–73.
[17] Rostand RA, Block AJ, Hunt L. Periodic sleep apnea: a family study of 3 cases. Chest 1978; 74:349.
[18] Redline S, Tishler PV, Tosteson TD, Williamson J, Kump K, Browner I, et al. The familial aggregation of obstructive sleep apnea. Am J Respir Crit Care Med 1995;151:682–7.
[19] Mathur R, Douglas NJ. Family studies in patients with the sleep apnea-hypopnea syndrome. Ann Intern Med 1995;122:174–8.

[20] Palmer LJ, Buxbaum SG, Larkin E, et al. A whole-genome scan for obstructive sleep apnea and obesity. Am J Hum Genet 2003;72:340–50.

[21] Jennum P, Hein HO, Suadicani P, et al. Snoring, family history, and genetic markers in men: the Copenhagen male study. Chest 1995;107:1289–93.

[22] Strohl KP, Hensley MJ, Hallett M, et al. Activation of upper airway muscles before onset of inspiration in normal humans. J Appl Physiol 1980;49:638–42.

[23] Suratt PM, McTier R, Wilhoit SC. Alae nasi electromyographic activity and timing in obstructive sleep apnea. J Appl Physiol 1985;58:1252–6.

[24] Yoshizawa T, Akashiba T, Kurashina K, et al. Genetics and obstructive sleep apnea syndrome: a study of human leukocyte antigen (HLA) typing. Intern Med 1993;32:94–7.

[25] Xiao Y, Huang X, Qiu C, et al. Angiotensin I-converting enzyme gene polymorphism in Chinese patients with obstructive sleep apnea syndrome. Chin Med J (Engl) 1999;112:701–4.

[26] Lin L, Finn L, Zhang J, et al. Angiotensin-converting enzyme, sleep-disordered breathing, and hypertension. Am J Respir Crit Care Med 2004;170:1349–53.

[27] Bliwise DL. Sleep apnea, APOE4 and Alzheimer's disease 20 years and counting? J Psychosom Res 2002;53:539–46.

[28] Kadotani H, Kadotani T, Young T, et al. Association between apolipoprotein E epsilon 4 and sleep-disordered breathing in adults. JAMA 2001;285(22):2888–90.

[29] Foley DJ, Masaki K, White L, et al. Sleep-disordered breathing and cognitive impairment in elderly Japanese-American men. Sleep 2003;26:596–9.

[30] Tishler PV, Larkin EK, Schluchter MD, et al. Incidence of sleep-disordered breathing in an urban adult population: the relative importance of risk factors in the development of sleep-disordered breathing. JAMA 2003;289:2230–7.

[31] Young T, Palta M, Dempsey J, et al. The occurrence of sleep-disordered breathing among middle-aged adults. N Engl J Med 1993;328:1230–5.

[32] Schwab RJ, Pasirstein M, Pierson R, et al. Identification of upper airway anatomic risk factors for obstructive sleep apnea with volumetric magnetic resonance imaging. Am J Respir Crit Care Med 2003;168:522–30.

[33] Despres JP, Lemieux I, Prudhomme D. Treatment of obesity: need to focus on high risk abdominally obese patients. BMJ 2001;322:716–20.

[34] Feitosa MF, Borecki I, Hunt SC, et al. Inheritance of the waist-to-hip ratio in the National Heart, Lung, and Blood Institute family heart study. Obes Res 2000;8:294–301.

[35] Bouchard C, Tremblay A, Despres JP, et al. The response to long-term overfeeding in identical twins. N Engl J Med 1990;322:1477–82.

[36] Chagnon YC, Rankinen T, Snyder EE, et al. The human obesity gene map: the 2002 update. Obes Res 2003;11:313–67.

[37] Loos RJ, Bouchard C. Obesity: is it a genetic disorder? J Intern Med 2003;254:401–25.

[38] Bluher S, Mantzoros CS. The role of leptin in regulating neuroendocrine function in humans. J Nutr 2004;134(Suppl):S2469–74.

[39] Montague CT, Farooqi IS, Whitehead JP, et al. Congenital leptin deficiency is associated with severe early-onset obesity in humans. Nature 1997;387:903–8.

[40] Farooqi IS, Jebb SA, Langmack G, et al. Effects of recombinant leptin therapy in a child with congenital leptin deficiency. N Engl J Med 1999;341:879–84.

[41] Considine RV, Sinha MK, Heiman ML, et al. Serum immunoreactive-leptin concentrations in normal-weight and obese humans. N Engl J Med 1996;334:292–5.

[42] Ozcelik O, Dogan H, Celik H, et al. Effects of different weight loss protocols on serum leptin levels in obese females. Physiol Res, in press.

[43] Couce ME, Green D, Brunetto A, et al. Limited brain access for leptin in obesity. Pituitary 2001; 4:101–10.

[44] Rohner-Jeanrenaud F, Jeanrenaud B. Obesity, leptin, and the brain. N Engl J Med 1996;334: 324–5.

[45] Livshits G, Pantsulaia I, Gerber LM. Association of leptin levels with obesity and blood pressure: possible common genetic variation. Int J Obes Relat Metab Disord 2005;29:85–92.

[46] Larkin EK, Elston RC, Patel SR, et al. Linkage of serum leptin levels in families with sleep apnea. Int J Obes Relat Metab Disord, in press.

[47] Rosenbaum M, Nicolson M, Hirsch J, et al. Effects of gender, body composition, and menopause on plasma concentrations of leptin. J Clin Endocrinol Metab 1996;81:3424–7.

[48] Schafer H, Pauleit D, Sudhop T, et al. Body fat distribution, serum leptin, and cardiovascular risk factors in men with obstructive sleep apnea. Chest 2002;122:829–39.

[49] Ip MS, Lam KS, Ho C, et al. Serum leptin and vascular risk factors in obstructive sleep apnea. Chest 2000;118:580–6.

[50] O'Donnell CP, Schaub CD, Haines AS, et al. Leptin prevents respiratory depression in obesity. Am J Respir Crit Care Med 1999;159:1477–84.

[51] Tankersley CG, O'Donnell C, Daood MJ, et al. Leptin attenuates respiratory complications associated with the obese phenotype. J Appl Physiol 1998;85:2261–9.

[52] Shioda S, Funahashi H, Nakajo S, et al. Immunohistochemical localization of leptin receptor in the rat brain. Neurosci Lett 1998;243:41–4.

[53] Chan JL, Bluher S, Yiannakouris N, et al. Regulation of circulating soluble leptin receptor levels by gender, adiposity, sex steroids, and leptin: observational and interventional studies in humans. Diabetes 2002;51:2105–12.

[54] Switonska MM, Kaczmarek P, Malendowicz LK, et al. Orexins and adipoinsular axis function in the rat. Regul Pept 2002;104:69–73.

[55] Sinton CM, Fitch TE, Gershenfeld HK. The effects of leptin on REM sleep and slow wave delta in rats are reversed by food deprivation. J Sleep Res 1999;8:197–203.

[56] Spiegel K, Tasali E, Penev P, et al. Sleep curtailment in healthy young men is associated with decreased leptin levels, elevated ghrelin levels, and increased hunger and appetite. Ann Intern Med 2004;141:846–50.

[57] Yoshimitsu N, Douchi T, Nagata Y. Perioperative changes in circulating leptin levels in women undergoing total abdominal hysterectomy. Endocr J 2001;48:509–13.

[58] Kain ZN, Zimolo Z, Heninger G. Leptin and the perioperative neuroendocrinological stress response. J Clin Endocrinol Metab 1999;84:2438–42.

[59] Miles PG, Vig PS, Weyant RJ, et al. Craniofacial structure and obstructive sleep apnea syndrome: a qualitative analysis and meta-analysis of the literature. Am J Orthod Dentofacial Orthop 1996;109:163–72.

[60] Li HY, Chen NH, Wang CR, et al. Use of 3-dimensional computed tomography scan to evaluate upper airway patency for patients undergoing sleep-disordered breathing surgery. Otolaryngol Head Neck Surg 2003;129:336–42.

[61] Jamieson A, Guilleminault C, Partinen M, et al. Obstructive sleep apneic patients have craniomandibular abnormalities. Sleep 1986;9:469–77.

[62] Kushida CA, Efron B, Guilleminault C. A predictive morphometric model for the obstructive sleep apnea syndrome. Ann Intern Med 1997;127:581–7.

[63] Tishler PV, Redline S, Ferrette V, et al. The association of sudden unexpected infant death with obstructive sleep apnea. Am J Respir Crit Care Med 1996;153:1857–63.

[64] Redline S, Tishler PV, Hans MG, et al. Racial differences in sleep-disordered breathing in African-Americans and Caucasians. Am J Respir Crit Care Med 1997;155:186–92.

[65] Osborne RH, DeGeorge FV. Genetic basis of morphologic variation: an evaluation and application of the twin study method. Cambridge: Harvard University Press; 1959.

[66] Lundstrom A. Nature versus nurture in dento-facial variation. Eur J Orthod 1984;6:77–91.

[67] Remmers JE, deGroot WJ, Sauerland EK, et al. Pathogenesis of upper airway occlusion during sleep. J Appl Physiol 1978;44:931–8.

[68] Georgopoulus D, Giannouli E, Tsara V, et al. Respiratory short-term poststimulus potentiation (after-discharge) in patients with obstructive sleep apnea. Am Rev Respir Dis 1992;146:1250–5.

[69] Tkacova R, Niroumand M, Lorenzi-Filho G, et al. Overnight shift from obstructive to central apneas in patients with heart failure: role of P_{CO_2} and circulatory delay. Circulation 2001;103:238–43.

[70] Kawakami Y, Yamamoto H, Yoshikawa T, et al. Chemical and behavioral control of breathing in adult twins. Am Rev Respir Dis 1984;129:703–7.

[71] Fleetham JA, Arnup ME, Anthonisen NR. Familial aspects of ventilatory control in patients with chronic obstructive pulmonary disease. Am Rev Respir Dis 1984;129:3–7.

[72] Beall CM, Strohl KP, Blangero J, et al. Quantitative genetic analysis of arterial oxygen saturation in Tibetan highlanders. Hum Biol 1997;69:597–604.

[73] Paton JY, Swaminathan S, Sargent CW, et al. Hypoxic and hypercapnic ventilatory responses in awake children with congenital central hypoventilation syndrome. Am Rev Respir Dis 1989;140: 368–72.

[74] Sasaki A, Kanai M, Kijima K, et al. Molecular analysis of congenital central hypoventilation syndrome. Hum Genet 2003;114:22–6.

[75] Redline S, Leitner J, Arnold J, et al. Ventilatory-control abnormalities in familial sleep apnea. Am J Respir Crit Care Med 1997;156:155–60.

[76] Hirshman CA, McCullough RE, Weil JV. Normal values for hypoxic and hypercapnic ventilatory drives in man. J Appl Physiol 1975;38:1095–8.

[77] Groeben H, Meier S, Tankersley CG, et al. Heritable differences in respiratory drive and breathing pattern in mice during anaesthesia and emergence. Br J Anaesth 2003;91:541–5.

[78] Groeben H, Meier S, Tankersley CG, et al. Influence of volatile anaesthetics on hypercapnoeic ventilatory responses in mice with blunted respiratory drive. Br J Anaesth 2004;92:697–703.

[79] Guilleminault C, Pelayo R. Narcolepsy. In: Kryger MH, Roth T, Dement WC, editors. Principles and practice of sleep medicine. Philadelphia: WB Saunders; 2000. p. 676–86.

[80] Nishino S, Okura M, Mignot E. Narcolepsy: genetic predisposition and neuropharmacological mechanisms. Sleep Med Rev 2000;4:57–99.

[81] Nishijima T, Sakurai S, Arihara Z, et al. Plasma orexin-A-like immunoreactivity in patients with sleep apnea hypopnea syndrome. Peptides 2003;24:407–11.

[82] Sakurai S, Nishijima T, Takahashi S, et al. Clinical significance of daytime plasma orexin-A-like immunoreactivity concentrations in patients with obstructive sleep apnea hypopnea syndrome. Respiration 2004;71:380–4.

[83] Busquets X, Barbe F, Barcelo A, et al. Decreased plasma levels of orexin-A in sleep apnea. Respiration 2004;71:575–9.

ELSEVIER
SAUNDERS

Anesthesiology Clin N Am
23 (2005) 463–478

ANESTHESIOLOGY
CLINICS OF
NORTH AMERICA

Preoperative Evaluation of Patients with Obesity and Obstructive Sleep Apnea

Rafael Cartagena, MD

Department of Anesthesiology, University of North Carolina School of Medicine, N2201, CB 7010, Chapel Hill, NC 27599-7010, USA

Obesity is a major public health concern in industrialized nations. In 2000 it was determined that almost 20% of US adults were obese [1]. Furthermore, it has been projected that this figure could double by 2025 [2]. Similar trends are developing worldwide, prompting the WHO to refer to obesity as a global epidemic [3]. Obesity is commonly defined as a body mass index (BMI) greater than 30 kg/m^2. A BMI greater than 35 kg/m^2 implies morbid obesity, and supermorbid obesity is defined by a BMI greater than 55 kg/m^2 [4]. Although obesity itself has been found to significantly decrease life expectancy [5], much of the morbidity and mortality of obesity is caused by other medical conditions that have been found to exist at increased rates in the obese population (Table 1). A strict causal relationship has not been established to link obesity with all of these conditions, but many of these comorbidities will improve with weight loss.

Obese individuals are a rapidly growing segment of the population and on average consume more health care resources than normal weight individuals [6,7]. Anesthesiologists should expect the perioperative care of obese patients to become an increasing portion of their practice. It is unclear whether there is an increased risk of perioperative complications in this population and what, if anything, can be done to reduce this risk. A large prospective trial [8] evaluating in-hospital surgical morbidity and mortality of obese patients compared with normal weight patients has revealed that the only statistically significant increase in complications seen in the obese population is wound infection. Although the authors stated that preoperative evaluation did not differ between obese and non-obese patients, there was no reference to anesthetic management. As a counter-

E-mail address: rcartagena@aims.unc.edu

Table 1
Conditions associated with obesity

Organ system	Conditions
Cardiovascular	Venous stasis, cerebral vascular accidents, pulmonary embolism, cardiomyopathy, arrhythmia, hypertension, hyperlipidemia, ischemic heart disease, peripheral vascular disease
Respiratory	Obstructive sleep apnea, obesity hypoventilation syndrome, sleep disordered breathing, restrictive respiratory impairment
Endocrine	Diabetes mellitus, hypothyroidism, Cushing's disease
Gastrointestinal	Cholelithiasis, gastroesophageal reflux disease, cirrhosis
Immunologic	Impaired immune response [79]
Musculoskeletal	Osteoarthritis, degenerative disk disease
Oncologic	Breast, colorectal, esophageal, kidney, endometrial cancers [80] and possibly others

Data from Adams JP, Murphy PG. Obesity in anesthesia and intensive care. Br J Anaesth 2000; 85(1):91–108.

point to these findings, there are a number of studies suggesting that obesity does increase the risk of perioperative respiratory complications [9–12], difficulty in airway management [13–15], and diminished perioperative cardiac function [16]. With this information in mind, it would appear that obesity does have the potential to increase the incidence of perioperative complications and that a careful preoperative assessment of these patients is likely to help reduce this risk. Despite this commonly held perception, to date there are no data indicating that preoperative assessment of obese patients has a positive impact on outcomes.

Obstructive sleep apnea (OSA) is the most common form of sleep-disordered breathing. In the United States, it has been estimated that 2% of middle-aged females and 4% of middle-aged males have OSA [17]. Conventional wisdom states that the majority of patients who suffer from OSA are undiagnosed and untreated [18]. These findings imply that a significant portion of OSA patients who present for surgery will not be diagnosed and that the anesthesiologist must screen patients suspected of having sleep-disordered breathing to customize the anesthetic care and begin necessary evaluations and therapy [19].

OSA can have a significant impact on the quality of life of affected patients. Recurrent episodes of apnea result in episodes of hypoxia, hypercapnia, and arousal, leading to an increase in sympathetic tone. Over time there is a significant impact on the cardiovascular system (Table 2) that can result in systemic and pulmonary hypertension, polycythemia, right- and left-sided heart failure, stroke, arrhythmias, and myocardial ischemia. Additionally, cognitive changes can occur because of repeated nocturnal arousal and inadequate deep stage and rapid eye movement (REM) sleep.

The perioperative care of patients with OSA will frequently involve challenges in airway management and cardiovascular compromise in more severe or long-standing cases. Despite these concerns, the diagnosis of OSA may not be an independent risk factor for perioperative complications in ambulatory surgery [20], and the role OSA plays in the morbidity and mortality of patients under-

Table 2
Pathophysiologic consequences of obstructive sleep apnea

Cardiovascular	Cognitive
Systemic hypertension	Hypersomnolence
Pulmonary hypertension	Personality changes
Polycythemia	Cognitive deficits
Right-sided heart failure	Accident prone
Left-sided heart failure	
Stroke	
Arrhythmia	
Myocardial ischemia	

Data from Refs. [81–83].

going more invasive procedures is unclear. Nonetheless, given the known association of OSA with multiple medical conditions, it seems reasonable to assume that preoperative treatment of OSA may improve surgical outcomes. In subsets of patients, OSA has been linked to an increased risk of perioperative arrhythmia [21], pulmonary complications, and prolonged hospital stays [22]. In addition, OSA is suspected of increasing the risk of perioperative myocardial infarctions [23,24]. Despite the inability to quantify the exact risk that OSA poses to a given patient, the goals of the preoperative assessment are to identify challenges in airway management and existing complications of OSA and to ensure that any underlying medical conditions have been treated before surgery, in an effort to minimize whatever risk may be present.

There is a strong relationship between obesity and OSA. Morbid obesity is a significant risk factor for the development of OSA, in which the majority of patients diagnosed with OSA have a BMI greater than 29 [25]; however, not all obese patients have OSA, and OSA patients can have a normal BMI. Because obesity and OSA are distinct diagnoses, the preoperative assessment of patients with obesity and OSA will be discussed separately, although some of the issues that arise are common to both disorders.

Preoperative assessment of the obese patient

Airway assessment

A thorough preoperative assessment of the obese patient's airway is required before commencing any anesthetic. Obesity has long been associated with difficult airway management, with the incidence of difficult intubation reported to be 15% in morbidly obese patients undergoing upper airway surgery [13]. Additionally, a nearly threefold increase (20.2% versus 7.6%, respectively) in difficult laryngoscopy has been noted among obese patients compared with subjects with a normal body mass index [15]. The magnitude of obesity does not necessarily correlate with difficulty in managing the airway. Recently, Brodsky et al [26] have found that neck circumference (measured at the level of the thyroid cartilage) and a high Mallampati score are more reliable predictors of difficult laryngoscopy than weight or BMI. With this information in mind, a thorough airway examination of the obese patient should include a measurement of neck circumference along with more traditional measures such as a Mallampati score, mouth opening, and evaluation of dentition, thyromental distance, and neck range of motion. Based on the data of Brodsky et al [26], a neck circumference of approximately 44 cm would imply a likelihood of problematic intubation slightly greater than the rate of difficulty in airway management seen in the general population. This risk increases to 35% in a patient with a 60-cm neck circumference [26].

The potential for difficult mask ventilation should also be considered during the preoperative visit. Obesity has been identified as an independent risk factor for difficult facemask ventilation. Increasing this risk would be findings such as the presence of a beard, lack of teeth, and history of snoring [27]. Large breasts and a central distribution of the patient's weight may also add to the challenge. Reviewing previous anesthetic charts and directly questioning the patient about a history of difficult airway management are essential. If there is a concern that facemask ventilation or intubation will be difficult, these issues should be discussed with the patient during the preoperative evaluation, and alternative approaches, such as awake fiber-optic intubation, should be presented. In the event that an awake approach to securing the airway is planned, a discussion in advance provides the added benefit of familiarizing the patient with the process and reducing the anxiety associated with the procedure.

Assessment of respiratory function

Obese patients are at risk of suffering from a number of respiratory derangements, including OSA, obesity-hypoventilation syndrome (OHS), and restrictive respiratory impairment. The increase in body mass also results in increased oxygen consumption and carbon dioxide production. With these issues in mind, it is not surprising that acute postoperative pulmonary events are twice as likely in obese patients compared with a nonobese population [9].

In obese patients without coexisting pulmonary disease, it is not unusual to find some alteration in their pulmonary function. Typically, this alteration is described as a restrictive respiratory impairment based on the results of spirometry. The expiratory reserve volume (ERV), functional residual capacity, and total lung capacity are all significantly reduced, as is the total respiratory compliance. If the ERV falls below the closing volume, intrapulmonary shunt and hypoxemia may result. The cause for these derangements is believed to be mechanical alterations related to the excess adipose tissue and increases in intra-abdominal pressure [28]. Generally, the higher the BMI, the more likely it is that pulmonary function will be affected. In morbidly obese patients, an increase in total respiratory resistance can be seen, which further adds to the work of breathing [29]. Despite these findings, spirometry as a screening test is of no added value in the preoperative evaluation of obese patients [30] and is indicated only if clinically significant coexisting disease is present, such as chronic obstructive pulmonary disease (COPD) or OHS. Along these lines, chest radiographs are also unlikely to provide useful information in this population in the absence of a specific indication.

OHS is defined by chronic daytime hypoxemia ($PCO_2 \leq 65$ mm Hg) and hypoventilation ($PCO_2 \geq 45$ mm Hg) in an obese patient without the diagnosis of COPD. This syndrome is believed frequently to refer to obese patients with OSA but, in fact, is a distinct syndrome, although many of the affected patients will also have the diagnosis of OSA [31]. Pickwickian patients suffer from both OSA and OHS. In more severe cases of OHS, patients develop pulmonary hypertension, right ventricular hypertrophy, and eventually right-sided heart failure. The exact mechanism that results in OHS is not clear, although an impaired central ventilatory drive, respiratory muscle inefficiency, and fatigue, as well as diminished respiratory system compliance are all believed to play a role [32].

The most reasonable approach to screening an obese patient for OHS is to check room air pulse oximetry. This approach is an easy, inexpensive, and noninvasive test for daytime hypoxemia. If the patient has an oxygen saturation level of less than 96%, further evaluation is warranted. Arterial blood gas analysis is necessary to document carbon dioxide retention and make the diagnosis of OHS. Polycythemia is another clue suggestive of chronic hypoxemia. Once the diagnosis is made, several further studies are indicated to assess the severity of disease and plan the anesthetic. An electrocardiogram may detect rhythm disturbances and screen for ventricular hypertrophy. Chest radiography may reveal cardiomegaly and atelectasis in advanced cases and exclude COPD or another pulmonary process as a contributor to the hypoventilation. Echocardiography is essential to evaluate cardiac hypertrophy, myocardial contractility, and the approximation of pulmonary artery pressures. Because of the patient's body habitus, transesophageal echocardiography may be necessary to obtain adequate windows.

With these data, the anesthesiologist is in a position to have an informed discussion with the patient about the increased perioperative risk of morbidity and mortality and work with other members of the patient's care team to determine whether any interventions should be initiated before surgery in an effort to minimize the risk of complications. Interventions may include pharmacologic treatment of arrhythmias or treatment of heart failure. Although weight loss can be effective [33], most patients will be unable to accomplish significant weight loss before surgery [34]. Patients with OHS may benefit from continuous positive airway pressure (CPAP) therapy. In obese patients with hypercapnia, a 2-week period of CPAP therapy has been shown to be effective in correcting their abnormal ventilatory drive [35]. Additionally, Kaneko et al [36] have shown that CPAP can improve cardiac function in patients with OSA, and there is a possibility that this benefit may also occur in OHS patients.

Assessment of the cardiovascular system

Obese patients are at increased risk of venous stasis, pulmonary embolism, hypertension, cerebral vascular accidents, cardiomyopathy, arrhythmia, and ischemic heart disease [37]. Perioperative pulmonary embolism is a major concern in obese patients. An increased incidence of venous stasis in obese patients [38,39], together with the fact that obesity is a significant risk factor for pulmonary embolism in the general population, [40] is the basis for this concern. An increased risk of perioperative thrombotic events has been shown to exist in bariatric surgery [41] as well as in obese patients undergoing lower-extremity orthopedic procedures [42], but this risk has not been clearly defined for a wider range of surgeries.

Identifying which obese patients are particularly at risk during a preoperative visit would allow for the initiation of prophylaxis before surgery. Venous stasis disease, BMI greater than 60, truncal obesity, OHS, OSA, a previous incidence of pulmonary embolism, and hypercoagulable states have been suggested as factors that increase the baseline risk of perioperative pulmonary embolism in obese patients after bariatric surgery [43]. These indicators may be useful in identifying which obese patients are at the highest risk of pulmonary embolism for a wider range of surgeries, but further study is needed. Once a patient has been identified as being at increased risk, deep venous thrombosis prophylaxis should be discussed with the surgeon.

Hypertension can be found in as many as 60% of obese patients [44]. Although the exact mechanism of hypertension in this population is not known, improvement has been shown to occur with weight loss [45]. Adequate non-invasive blood pressure monitoring can be problematic in many obese patients. Examining and noting the general size and shape (cone or cylinder) of the patient's upper arm will assist in determining what size blood pressure cuff will be needed or whether invasive monitoring will be necessary. Performing this assessment preoperatively will assure that the operating room is properly equipped before the patient's arrival and avoid the possibility of embarrassing the patient because the cuff will not fit.

Obtaining a recent ECG as part of the preoperative evaluation is highly advisable. Despite excess adipose tissue present in the chest, which might be expected to produce a low-voltage ECG, this finding is present only in approximately 4% of obese individuals [46,47]. If present, a low-voltage ECG may obscure signs of left ventricular hypertrophy based on voltage criteria. Other findings may include axis deviation that worsens with increasing BMI, ST segment and T-wave abnormalities [46] and left atrial enlargement [48]. Obesity by itself does not appear to significantly increase the risk of conduction abnormalities [46], but arrhythmias may be present for a number of reasons, including OSA, OHS, coronary artery disease (CAD), myocardial hypertrophy, or atrial dilation. In the event the patient has cor pulmonale, signs of right ventricle hypertrophy may be present and include right-axis deviation and tall precordial R waves.

Because of the increased incidence of coronary artery disease and myocardial infarction in this population, the preoperative ECG is also helpful in providing a reference for comparison in the event that myocardial ischemia is suspected in the perioperative period. Beyond this consideration, there is no reason to believe that extensive preoperative testing to detect CAD is indicated based solely on a patient being obese [49]. Studies such as stress testing and echocardiography are best reserved for patients with a history and physical examination that suggest abnormalities and those who are undergoing high-risk surgical procedures. Symptoms and signs of heart failure such as exertional dyspnea, fatigue, peripheral edema, increased jugular venous distension, hepatomegaly, and pulmonary crackles can be used to screen for congestive heart failure. These findings may be difficult to detect in this population, but their presence should be investigated before ordering echocardiography to rule out congestive heart failure.

Other considerations

Obesity is significantly related to gastroesophageal reflux disease (GERD) [50]. Increased body mass has been shown to correlate directly with an increased incidence of reflux symptoms [51,52]. This evidence implies that during the preoperative assessment, all obese patients should be questioned directly regarding the presence of reflux symptoms. Some experts have stated that all obese patients are at increased risk of aspiration regardless of whether they report symptoms of GERD [53]. This conservative approach is based on the assumption that some obese patients will have GERD, confirmed objectively by pH measurement and esophageal monometry, yet are asymptomatic [54]. If symptoms are present or the conservative approach (assuming all obese patients have GERD) is chosen, the potentially increased risk of aspiration should be discussed with the patient, and prophylactic measures (cricoid pressure, H2 blockers, and proton pump inhibitors) should be considered. Although it is unclear which if any of these measures are effective [55], they are within the current standard of care. There is no consensus on whether obese patients have delayed, normal, or accelerated gastric emptying [56,57]. Given the uncertainty surrounding this issue, it would seem reasonable to require obese patients to follow the same "nothing-by-mouth" guidelines as nonobese patients before being anesthetized.

Adequate intravenous access is frequently difficult to obtain in obese patients. Evaluating the patient's peripheral vasculature will provide the opportunity to discuss with the patient any possible need for central venous access and to ensure that any necessary equipment for the placement of a central venous catheter, such as an ultrasonographic device, is available in the operating room on the patient's arrival.

The use of regional anesthetic techniques in obese patients offers many advantages, including safer postoperative analgesia [13,58] and avoiding airway manipulation. Unfortunately, excess body fat masks landmarks and makes regional anesthetic procedures more difficult in obese patients [53]. An evaluation of the landmarks necessary to provide a regional anesthetic appropriate for a given procedure should be performed during any preoperative visit. This can alert the anesthesiologist to the feasibility of a technique as well as to allow adequate time to arrange for any equipment and expertise needed to facilitate the procedure because of obscured landmarks. Examples would include fluoroscopy or ultrasonography [59] for epidural placement as well as ultrasonography and nerve stimulators for peripheral nerve blocks.

Finally, the preoperative assessment should include some consideration of the appropriateness of administering an anesthetic to a patient at the planned location. Morbid obesity is commonly believed to be a contraindication to performing procedures at an ambulatory surgery center (ASC). This belief is based on the reportedly increased risk of respiratory and other perioperative complications that would increase the likelihood that a postoperative admission would be required. A retrospective study by Davies et al [60] suggests that this may not be the case. These investigators found that morbid obesity (BMI ≥ 35 kg/m^2) alone did not significantly affect the rate of unplanned admissions or postoperative complications. Notably, the charts of all of the morbidly obese patients in this study were reviewed by an anesthesiologist who cleared the patients to undergo the procedures at the ASC; however, no mention was made of how many morbidly obese patients were diverted to a hospital-based operating room by the anesthesiologists during the study period or what criteria were used to guide these decisions. Further research into the necessity of this common practice is needed. As the population becomes more obese and nonhospital-based operating rooms accommodate an increasing volume of procedures, it is likely that assigning arbitrary patient weight limitations to these sites will be impractical without scientific justification, and this evidence does not yet exist.

Preoperative assessment of patients with obstructive sleep apnea

Identifying patients with obstructive sleep apnea

Many patients with OSA are undiagnosed [18], and identifying these individuals before the administration of an anesthetic is essential to delivering the highest standard of care. Directed questioning is an efficient and inexpensive means of screening patients for sleep-disordered breathing. In 2003, the clinical practice review committee of the American Academy of Sleep Medicine suggested a series of questions to assist in the screening for OSA (Box 1) as well as a list of findings suggestive of OSA (Box 2). Used in combination, these tools provide a means of determining who should be screened for OSA and what questions to ask. The presence of the patient's bedroom partner will increase the likelihood of accurately detecting symptoms suggestive of OSA because many of the questions in Box 1 refer to external observations of the patient. It is also important to note that not all patients with OSA will be detected by questioning and the reliability of such questionnaires has not been validated [19,61]. Other

---

Box 1. Questions for exploring obstructive sleep apnea symptoms

Do people tell you that you snore?
Do you wake up at night with a feeling of shortness of breath
  or choking?
Do people tell you that you gasp, choke, or snort while sleeping?
Do people tell you that you stop breathing while sleeping?
Do you awake feeling almost as or more tired than when you
  went to bed?
Do you often awake with a headache?
Do you often have difficulty breathing through your nose?
Do you fight sleepiness during the daytime?
Do you fall asleep when relaxing after meals?
Do others comment on your sleepiness during the day?

Data from Meoli AL, Rosen CL, Kristo D, et al. Upper airway
management of the adult patient with obstructive sleep apnea
in the perioperative period–avoiding complications. Sleep 2003;
26(8):1060–5.

---

clues that a patient may have OSA are unexplained polycythemia, room air hypoxemia, or signs of right-sided heart failure. Despite the lack of validation for these screening tools, there is no superior approach available currently to screen patients for OSA.

Once a patient who is suspected of having OSA is identified, the next step is to decide what, if anything, needs to be done before proceeding to the operating room. If the procedure is nonurgent, scheduling an evaluation by a sleep specialist to determine the need for a diagnostic sleep study before surgery is reasonable. There are several advantages to this approach. First, a formal diagnosis of OSA will most likely result in the initiation of CPAP therapy. This

---

Box 2. Findings that increase the risk that a patient suffers from obstructive sleep apnea

Gender: male
BMI greater than 25 kg/m^2
Neck circumference greater than 16 inches in females or greater
  than 17 inches in males [19]
Habitual snoring and gasping noted by bed partner
Daytime sleepiness
Hypertension
High Mallampati score [67]

---

therapy will allow for properly fitting the device and titration of the level of CPAP required, which can be difficult in the postoperative period. The patient also will be more likely to tolerate CPAP therapy in the perioperative period, if it should it be required to maintain airway patency under conditions of narcotic analgesics use or postoperative REM sleep rebound. Additionally, applying nasal CPAP to patients with OSA during propofol anesthesia has been shown to counteract airway closure [62], making nasal CPAP helpful in cases in which the anesthesiologist would prefer to avoid instrumenting the airway. Another advantage is that improvement in some cardiovascular sequelae of OSA can be seen within several weeks of initiating CPAP therapy [36,63]. A final potential benefit is that 4 to 6 weeks of CPAP therapy has been shown on magnetic resonance imaging to decrease tongue volume and increase pharyngeal in patients with OSA [64]. These changes may reduce the risk of encountering a difficult airway [65]. The most significant disadvantage in delaying surgery to formally diagnose and treat OSA is the relative difficulty of obtaining polysomnography in some regions, as well as the cost of the study. A quicker and less expensive way to detect OSA is to use one of the home-based testing systems currently available. Unfortunately, these systems have increased failure rates and are unable to detect the stage of sleep that a patient is in when an event occurs because the systems do not include an electroencephalogram [66].

Assessment of the patient with known obstructive sleep apnea

OSA and difficult intubation have been shown to be significantly related [67], which makes a thorough airway evaluation particularly importance when preparing to anesthetize a patient who has OSA. Measuring a patient's neck circumference is a worthwhile activity because a larger circumference is associated with an increasing severity of OSA [68] and difficult laryngoscopy [26]. A thorough airway assessment, however, will not always detect excess pharyngeal tissue, which may result in difficulty in managing the airway [69]. Regardless of the approach to airway management chosen by the anesthesia care team, the increased incidence of GERD found in this population [70] must be kept in mind, and the patient should be questioned about symptoms of reflux disease during the interview.

The primary treatment of moderate to severe OSA is nasal CPAP. Some milder cases may be responsive to conservative therapy, which includes weight loss, alcohol and smoking cessation, or changes in sleeping position, and the use of oral appliances. Patients with mild OSA who fail conservative management also may be placed on CPAP therapy, although compliance in this population is more problematic [71]. Asking a patient about what therapies they currently have been prescribed and assessing their compliance with these therapies are important parts of the preoperative interview. Postponing surgery for the noncompliant patient in an effort to optimize therapy and potentially reduce the risks of difficult airway management [64,65] and perioperative respiratory embarrassment [72] or to improve cardiovascular function [36,63] is a reasonable approach.

A frank discussion of the risks associated with the administration of an anesthetic to patients with significant OSA may be all the motivation that is required to improve compliance with CPAP therapy.

Cardiovascular consequences of obstructive sleep apnea

Patients with OSA are at risk of developing cardiovascular derangements as a result of increased sympathetic tone. Ascertaining whether any comorbidities are present and to what extent they are being treated is fundamental to preparing this population for surgery. Moderate and severe OSA are risk factors for developing systemic hypertension [73], and effective CPAP therapy has been shown to reduce arterial blood pressure [63]. Many hypertensive sleep apnea patients are still likely to require pharmacologic management of their blood pressure to approach normal values, and these medications should be continued in the perioperative period.

Pulmonary hypertension is another possible consequence of the repeated hypoxemia and hypercarbia that occur in OSA patients. This finding is more likely in patients with coexisting COPD or obesity hypoventilation syndrome. Although 15% to 20% of OSA patients will present with pulmonary hypertension, the severity of OSA does not necessarily correlate with worsening pulmonary hypertension [74]. Chronic daytime hypoxemia is a better predictor of right-sided heart failure and pulmonary hypertension than the severity of OSA as determined by polysomnography [75]. Based on these findings, the use of awake pulse oximetry readings as a screening tool for pulmonary hypertension in OSA patients is both practical and cost effective. If daytime hypoxemia is detected, then further evaluations, including arterial blood gas analysis and echocardiography, would be indicated to quantify the severity of hypoxemia and pulmonary hypertension as well as any affect on the right side of the heart. Notable, the majority of OSA patients with pulmonary hypertension will be found to have mild to moderate increases in pulmonary pressures and not require aggressive interventions or monitoring in the perioperative period [74]. Having OSA increases a person's risk of developing congestive heart failure (CHF) [76]. In patients with both OSA and CHF, the administration of CPAP therapy for 4 weeks resulted in a 35% relative increase in ejection fraction and a decrease in systemic blood pressure and heart rate [36]. Based on this data, it would appear likely that strict compliance to prescribed CPAP therapy would be an essential step in minimizing perioperative cardiac morbidity and mortality in this population, and surgery should be postponed, if possible, to allow this therapy to occur. Unfortunately, there is currently no evidence that the initiation of CPAP therapy reduces perioperative cardiac complications in this or any other population, and further study is clearly required.

OSA has been reported as an independent risk factor for myocardial ischemia [23,77]. To date there are no data to suggest that patients with OSA are at increased risk of perioperative myocardial infarction compared with all patients with coronary artery disease, but the increased risk of hypoxic events in the perioperative period could increase the odds of an unfavorable oxygen supply-to-demand relationship occurring perioperatively. All patients with suspected or known coronary artery disease should undergo an evaluation such as that suggested by the American Heart Association/American College of Cardiology guidelines for preoperative evaluation of a cardiac patient for non-cardiac surgery [78].

Summary

Obesity is a complex disorder that affects most organ systems directly or indirectly. Although management of the airway can be challenging in this population, a thorough preoperative visit provides the opportunity to plan appropriately and educate the patient about the risks and advantages of the chosen approach. Coexisting pulmonary and cardiovascular issues also must be identified and taken into consideration when planning the anesthetic. A final goal of the preoperative visit is to assess any potential impact that the patient's body habitus may have on technical issues such as positioning, availability of equipment, and location in which the procedure will be performed.

The key to providing the highest standard of care to patients with obstructive sleep apnea is the knowledge that the patient has this disease before initiating an anesthetic. Directed questioning about symptoms suggestive of OSA is a critical component of the preoperative evaluation in all patients that raise an index of suspicion. Delaying surgery to allow for a formal diagnosis and the initiation of therapy in suspected patients are advisable in all but the most urgent or non-invasive procedures. Assuring the optimization of CPAP therapy before surgery will minimize whatever risk of respiratory or cardiovascular complications may exist in this population.

References

[1] Mokdad AH, Bowman BA, Ford ES, et al. The continuing epidemics of obesity and diabetes in the United States. JAMA 2001;286(10):1195–200.

[2] Kopelman PG. Obesity as a medical problem. Nature 2000;404(6778):635–43.

[3] World Health Organization. Obesity-preventing and managing a global epidemic: report of the WHO consultation on obesity. Geneva: WHO; 1997.

[4] Bray GA. Pathophysiology of obesity. Am J Clin Nutr 1992;55(Suppl2):S488–94.

[5] Fontaine KR, Redden DT, Wang C, et al. Years of life lost due to obesity. JAMA 2003; 289(2):187–93.

[6] Thompson D, Wolf AM. The medical-care cost burden of obesity. Obes Rev 2001;2(3):189–97.

[7] Quesenberry Jr CP, Caan B, Jacobson A. Obesity, health services use, and health care costs among members of a health maintenance organization. Arch Intern Med 1998;158(5):466–72.

[8] Dindo D, Muller MK, Weber M, et al. Obesity in general elective surgery. Lancet 2003; 361(9374):2032–5.

[9] Rose DK, Cohen MM, Wigglesworth DF, et al. Critical respiratory events in the postanesthesia care unit: patient, surgical, and anesthetic factors. Anesthesiology 1994;81(2):410–8.

[10] Chung F, Mezei G, Tong D. Pre-existing medical conditions as predictors of adverse events in day-case surgery. Br J Anaesth 1999;83(2):262–70.

[11] Duncan PG, Cohen MM, Tweed WA, et al. The Canadian four-centre study of anaesthetic outcomes: III. are anaesthetic complications predictable in day surgical practice? Can J Anaesth 1992;39(5 Pt 1):440–8.

[12] Fleming ST. Outcomes of care for anesthesia services: a pilot study. Qual Assur Health Care 1992;4(4):289–303.

[13] Buckley FP, Robinson NB, Simonowitz DA, et al. Anaesthesia in the morbidly obese: a comparison of anaesthetic and analgesic regimens for upper abdominal surgery. Anaesthesia 1983; 38(9):840–51.

[14] Hood DD, Dewan DM. Anesthetic and obstetric outcome in morbidly obese parturients. Anesthesiology 1993;79(6):1210–8.

[15] Voyagis GS, Kyriakis KP, Dimitriou V, et al. Value of oropharyngeal Mallampati classification in predicting difficult laryngoscopy among obese patients. Eur J Anaesthesiol 1998;15(3):330–4.

[16] Agarwal N, Shibutani K, SanFilippo JA, et al. Hemodynamic and respiratory changes in surgery of the morbidly obese. Surgery 1982;92(2):226–34.

[17] Young T, Palta M, Dempsey J, et al. The occurrence of sleep-disordered breathing among middle-aged adults. N Engl J Med 1993;328(17):1230–5.

[18] Young T, Evans L, Finn L, et al. Estimation of the clinically diagnosed proportion of sleep apnea syndrome in middle-aged men and women. Sleep 1997;20(9):705–6.

[19] Meoli AL, Rosen CL, Kristo D, et al. Upper airway management of the adult patient with obstructive sleep apnea in the perioperative period–avoiding complications. Sleep 2003;26(8): 1060–5.

[20] Sabers C, Plevak DJ, Schroeder DR, et al. The diagnosis of obstructive sleep apnea as a risk factor for unanticipated admissions in outpatient surgery. Anesth Analg 2003;96(5):1328–35 [table of contents].

[21] Mooe T, Gullsby S, Rabben T, et al. Sleep-disordered breathing: a novel predictor of atrial fibrillation after coronary artery bypass surgery. Coron Artery Dis 1996;7(6):475–8.

[22] Gupta RM, Parvizi J, Hanssen AD, et al. Postoperative complications in patients with obstructive sleep apnea syndrome undergoing hip or knee replacement: a case-control study. Mayo Clin Proc 2001;76(9):897–905.

[23] Hung J, Whitford EG, Parsons RW, et al. Association of sleep apnoea with myocardial infarction in men. Lancet 1990;336(8710):261–4.

[24] Dominguez Ortega L, Carnevali-Ruiz D, Diaz Gallego E. Sleep apnea and the risk for perioperative myocardial infarction. Ann Intern Med 1993;119(9):953.

[25] Strohl KP, Redline S. Recognition of obstructive sleep apnea. Am J Respir Crit Care Med 1996;154(2 Pt 1):279–89.

[26] Brodsky JB, Lemmens HJ, Brock-Utne JG, et al. Morbid obesity and tracheal intubation. Anesth Analg 2002;94(3):732–6 [table of contents].

[27] Langeron O, Masso E, Huraux C, et al. Prediction of difficult mask ventilation. Anesthesiology 2000;92(5):1229–36.

[28] Pelosi P, Croci M, Ravagnan I, et al. Respiratory system mechanics in sedated, paralyzed, morbidly obese patients. J Appl Physiol 1997;82(3):811–8.

[29] Pelosi P, Croci M, Ravagnan I, et al. The effects of body mass on lung volumes, respiratory mechanics, and gas exchange during general anesthesia. Anesth Analg 1998;87(3):654–60.

[30] Crapo RO, Kelly TM, Elliott CG, et al. Spirometry as a preoperative screening test in morbidly obese patients. Surgery 1986;99(6):763–8.

[31] Kessler R, Chaouat A, Schinkewitch P, et al. The obesity-hypoventilation syndrome revisited: a prospective study of 34 consecutive cases. Chest 2001;120(2):369–76.

[32] Koenig SM. Pulmonary complications of obesity. Am J Med Sci 2001;321(4):249–79.

[33] Oxorn DC, Dauphinee KR, Vincent G. Partial reversal of the obesity hypoventilation syndrome with weight reduction. Anaesth Intensive Care 1988;16(2):224–7.

[34] Coe AJ, Saleh T, Samuel T, et al. The management of patients with morbid obesity in the anaesthetic assessment clinic. Anaesthesia 2004;59(6):570–3.

[35] Lin CC. Effect of nasal CPAP on ventilatory drive in normocapnic and hypercapnic patients with obstructive sleep apnoea syndrome. Eur Respir J 1994;7(11):2005–10.

[36] Kaneko Y, Floras JS, Usui K, et al. Cardiovascular effects of continuous positive airway pressure in patients with heart failure and obstructive sleep apnea. N Engl J Med 2003;348(13): 1233–41.

[37] Hubert HB, Feinleib M, McNamara PM, et al. Obesity as an independent risk factor for cardiovascular disease: a 26-year follow-up of participants in the Framingham Heart Study. Circulation 1983;67(5):968–77.

[38] Kakkar VV, Howe CT, Nicolaides AN, et al. Deep vein thrombosis of the leg: is there a "high risk" group? Am J Surg 1970;120(4):527–30.

[39] Clayton JK, Anderson JA, McNicol GP. Preoperative prediction of postoperative deep vein thrombosis. BMJ 1976;2(6041):910–2.

[40] Goldhaber SZ, Grodstein F, Stampfer MJ, et al. A prospective study of risk factors for pulmonary embolism in women. JAMA 1997;277(8):642–5.

[41] Martin Jr EW, Mojzisik C, Carey LC. Complications of gastric restrictive operations in morbidly obese patients. Surg Clin North Am 1983;63(6):1181–90.

[42] Mantilla CB, Horlocker TT, Schroeder DR, et al. Risk factors for clinically relevant pulmonary embolism and deep venous thrombosis in patients undergoing primary hip or knee arthroplasty. Anesthesiology 2003;99(3):552–60 [discussion 555A].

[43] Sapala JA, Wood MH, Schuhknecht MP, et al. Fatal pulmonary embolism after bariatric operations for morbid obesity: a 24-year retrospective analysis. Obes Surg 2003;13(6): 819–25.

[44] Alexander JK. Obesity and cardiac performance. Am J Cardiol 1964;14:860–5.

[45] Alpert MA, Lambert CR, Panayiotou H, et al. Relation of duration of morbid obesity to left ventricular mass, systolic function, and diastolic filling, and effect of weight loss. Am J Cardiol 1995;76(16):1194–7.

[46] Frank S, Colliver JA, Frank A. The electrocardiogram in obesity: statistical analysis of 1,029 patients. J Am Coll Cardiol 1986;7(2):295–9.

[47] Eisenstein I, Edelstein J, Sarma R, et al. The electrocardiogram in obesity. J Electrocardiol 1982;15(2):115–8.

[48] Alpert MA, Terry BE, Cohen MV, et al. The electrocardiogram in morbid obesity. Am J Cardiol 2000;85(7):908–10 [discussion A910].

[49] Ramaswamy A, Gonzalez R, Smith CD. Extensive preoperative testing is not necessary in morbidly obese patients undergoing gastric bypass. J Gastrointest Surg 2004;8(2):159–64.

[50] Murray L, Johnston B, Lane A, et al. Relationship between body mass and gastro-oesophageal reflux symptoms: the Bristol Helicobacter Project. Int J Epidemiol 2003;32(4):645–50.

[51] Nilsson M, Johnsen R, Ye W, et al. Obesity and estrogen as risk factors for gastroesophageal reflux symptoms. JAMA 2003;290(1):66–72.

[52] Fisher BL, Pennathur A, Mutnick JL, et al. Obesity correlates with gastroesophageal reflux. Dig Dis Sci 1999;44(11):2290–4.

[53] Adams JP, Murphy PG. Obesity in anaesthesia and intensive care. Br J Anaesth 2000;85(1): 91–108.

[54] Suter M, Dorta G, Giusti V, et al. Gastro-esophageal reflux and esophageal motility disorders in morbidly obese patients. Obes Surg 2004;14(7):959–66.

[55] Kalinowski CP, Kirsch JR. Strategies for prophylaxis and treatment for aspiration. Best Pract Res Clin Anaesthesiol 2004;18(4):719–37.

[56] Jackson SJ, Leahy FE, McGowan AA, et al. Delayed gastric emptying in the obese: an assessment using the non-invasive (13)C-octanoic acid breath test. Diabetes Obes Metab 2004;6(4): 264–70.

[57] Verdich C, Madsen JL, Toubro S, et al. Effect of obesity and major weight reduction on gastric emptying. Int J Obes Relat Metab Disord 2000;24(7):899–905.

[58] Shenkman Z, Shir Y, Brodsky JB. Perioperative management of the obese patient. Br J Anaesth 1993;70(3):349–59.

[59] Wallace DH, Currie JM, Gilstrap LC, et al. Indirect sonographic guidance for epidural anesthesia in obese pregnant patients. Reg Anesth 1992;17(4):233–6.

[60] Davies KE, Houghton K, Montgomery JE. Obesity and day-case surgery. Anaesthesia 2001; 56(11):1112–5.

[61] Kump K, Whalen C, Tishler PV, et al. Assessment of the validity and utility of a sleep-symptom questionnaire. Am J Respir Crit Care Med 1994;150(3):735–41.

[62] Mathru M, Esch O, Lang J, et al. Magnetic resonance imaging of the upper airway: effects of propofol anesthesia and nasal continuous positive airway pressure in humans. Anesthesiology 1996;84(2):273–9.

[63] Becker HF, Jerrentrup A, Ploch T, et al. Effect of nasal continuous positive airway pressure treatment on blood pressure in patients with obstructive sleep apnea. Circulation 2003;107(1): 68–73.

[64] Ryan CF, Lowe AA, Li D, et al. Magnetic resonance imaging of the upper airway in obstructive sleep apnea before and after chronic nasal continuous positive airway pressure therapy. Am Rev Respir Dis 1991;144(4):939–44.

[65] Mehta Y, Manikappa S, Juneja R, et al. Obstructive sleep apnea syndrome: anesthetic implications in the cardiac surgical patient. J Cardiothorac Vasc Anesth 2000;14(4):449–53.

[66] Baumel MJ, Maislin G, Pack AI. Population and occupational screening for obstructive sleep apnea: are we there yet? Am J Respir Crit Care Med 1997;155(1):9–14.

[67] Hiremath AS, Hillman DR, James AL, et al. Relationship between difficult tracheal intubation and obstructive sleep apnoea. Br J Anaesth 1998;80(5):606–11.

[68] Katz I, Stradling J, Slutsky AS, et al. Do patients with obstructive sleep apnea have thick necks? Am Rev Respir Dis 1990;141(5 Pt 1):1228–31.

[69] Benumof JL. Obstructive sleep apnea in the adult obese patient: implications for airway management. J Clin Anesth 2001;13(2):144–56.

[70] Gislason T, Janson C, Vermeire P, et al. Respiratory symptoms and nocturnal gastroesophageal reflux: a population-based study of young adults in three European countries. Chest 2002; 121(1):158–63.

[71] Grunstein RR. Sleep-related breathing disorders. 5. Nasal continuous positive airway pressure treatment for obstructive sleep apnoea. Thorax 1995;50(10):1106–13.

[72] Rennotte MT, Baele P, Aubert G, et al. Nasal continuous positive airway pressure in the perioperative management of patients with obstructive sleep apnea submitted to surgery. Chest 1995;107(2):367–74.

[73] Peppard PE, Young T, Palta M, et al. Prospective study of the association between sleep-disordered breathing and hypertension. N Engl J Med 2000;342(19):1378–84.

[74] Kessler R, Chaouat A, Weitzenblum E, et al. Pulmonary hypertension in the obstructive sleep apnoea syndrome: prevalence, causes and therapeutic consequences. Eur Respir J 1996;9(4): 787–94.

[75] Bradley TD, Rutherford R, Grossman RF, et al. Role of daytime hypoxemia in the pathogenesis of right heart failure in the obstructive sleep apnea syndrome. Am Rev Respir Dis 1985; 131(6):835–9.

[76] Shahar E, Whitney CW, Redline S, et al. Sleep-disordered breathing and cardiovascular disease: cross-sectional results of the Sleep Heart Health Study. Am J Respir Crit Care Med 2001; 163(1):19–25.

[77] Koskenvuo M, Kaprio J, Heikkila K, et al. Snoring as a risk factor for ischaemic heart disease and stroke in men. BMJ 1987;294(6572):643.

[78] Eagle KA, Berger PB, Calkins H, et al. ACC/AHA guideline update for perioperative cardiovascular evaluation for noncardiac surgery–executive summary: a report of the American College of Cardiology/American Heart Association Task Force on practice guidelines (committee to update the 1996 guidelines on perioperative cardiovascular evaluation for noncardiac surgery). Anesth Analg 2002;94(5):1052–64.

[79] Tanaka S, Inoue S, Isoda F, et al. Impaired immunity in obesity: suppressed but reversible lymphocyte responsiveness. Int J Obes Relat Metab Disord 1993;17(11):631–6.

[80] Calle EE, Thun MJ. Obesity and cancer. Oncogene 2004;23(38):6365–78.

[81] Shepard Jr JW. Hypertension, cardiac arrhythmias, myocardial infarction, and stroke in relation to obstructive sleep apnea. Clin Chest Med 1992;13(3):437–58.

[82] Partinen M, Jamieson A, Guilleminault C. Long-term outcome for obstructive sleep apnea syndrome patients: mortality. Chest 1988;94(6):1200–4.

[83] Mooe T, Franklin KA, Holmstrom K, et al. Sleep-disordered breathing and coronary artery disease: long-term prognosis. Am J Respir Crit Care Med 2001;164(10 Pt 1):1910–3.

ELSEVIER
SAUNDERS

Anesthesiology Clin N Am
23 (2005) 479–491

ANESTHESIOLOGY
CLINICS OF
NORTH AMERICA

Anesthetic Management of Patients with Obesity and Sleep Apnea

Anthony N. Passannante, MD*,
Peter Rock, MD, MBA, FCCP, FCCM

Department of Anesthesiology, University of North Carolina School of Medicine, N2201, CB 7010, Chapel Hill, NC 27599-7010, USA

Obesity has become one of the most important public health problems confronting industrialized nations. Recent data demonstrate that more than 30% of the US population is obese (body mass index [BMI] ≥30) and 4.9% of the population is morbidly obese (BMI ≥40) [1]. Because many chronic health problems such as cardiovascular disease, diabetes mellitus, arthritis, and cancer are associated with obesity, it is certain that anesthesiologists are going to care for an increasing number of obese patients for the foreseeable future. Given recent reports [2] that indicate that bariatric surgery offers sustained reductions in body weight and reductions in cardiovascular risk factors, it is likely that laparoscopic gastric bypass surgery will bring an increasing number of obese patients to the operating room. A recent report [3] suggests that bariatric surgery reduces overall mortality. The first section of this article concentrates on intraoperative issues in patients with obesity, and airway management is covered elsewhere. The major topics to be covered are the pharmacokinetics of obesity, positioning of obese patients, regional anesthesia, the intensity of monitoring required, laparoscopy, and minimizing hypoxia during anesthesia.

Pharmacokinetics of obesity

As with normal weight patients, the main factors that affect tissue drug distribution in obese patients are plasma protein binding, body composition, and

---

* Corresponding author.
E-mail address: apassannante@aims.unc.edu (A.N. Passannante).

0889-8537/05/$ – see front matter © 2005 Elsevier Inc. All rights reserved.
doi:10.1016/j.atc.2005.02.005
anesthesiology.theclinics.com

regional blood flow. Changes in any of these factors may alter the volume of distribution of a drug. Although plasma protein binding has not been studied extensively, it does not appear to be significantly different in obese individuals. Obese patients do have both an increased lean body mass (LBM) and an increased fat mass, but the percentage of increase in fat mass is greater than the percentage of increase in lean body mass [4]. Simple mathematics leads to the conclusion that obese patients will thus have less lean body mass per kilogram and more fat body mass per kilogram than normal weight individuals will. Under usual circumstances, blood flow to fat is poor, accounting for perhaps 5% of cardiac output, compared with approximately 73% to viscera and 22% to lean tissue [5]. Because blood volume increases directly with body weight, and many obese individuals will have an increased cardiac output, the vessel-rich group of organs is well perfused in obese individuals [6,7]. This has implications for both injected and inhaled anesthetics. Unfortunately, the obesity pandemic has not given rise to an increase in pharmacokinetic studies in obese patients. Data regarding four classes of anesthetic drugs are summarized: induction drugs (unfortunately, only propofol), opioids, neuromuscular blockers, and volatile anesthetics.

Because of many factors, including its favorable early recovery profile, pharmacokinetic studies of induction drugs have concentrated on propofol. A comparison study [8] with normal weight controls showed that administering doses of propofol on the basis of total body weight (TBW) gave acceptable clinical results, unchanged initial volume of distribution, and clearance related to body weight and that the volume of distribution at steady state was correlated with body weight. There was no evidence of propofol accumulation when dosing schemes based on mg/kg of total body weight were used.

The situation is somewhat more complicated with regard to opioids. The pharmacokinetics of remifentanil of 12 obese patients were compared with 12 normal weight control subjects [9], and the obese subjects reached significantly higher plasma concentrations after a loading dose than the normal subjects, suggesting that to avoid an overdose, remifentanil should be administered on the basis of ideal body weight (IBW) or LBM. Although sufentanil is not extensively used in current clinical practice, a recent study [10] measured plasma sufentanil levels during and after an infusion, directed by parameters derived from a normal weight population (as virtually all drug dosage recommendations are derived), and found that the actual plasma concentrations of sufentanil were accurately predicted when dosing was based on TBW. With the more commonly administered opioid fentanyl, a different relationship exists. Another recent study [11] compared the plasma concentrations of fentanyl measured in normal (BMI ≤30) and obese (BMI ≥30) subjects undergoing major surgery with a fentanyl infusion based on TBW and found that such an infusion led to an overestimation of fentanyl dose requirements in obese patients. The authors derived a parameter they refer to as pharmacokinetic mass, which could be used to linearly predict fentanyl clearance and thus accurately guide fentanyl infusions. For patients weighing 140 to 200 kg, the pharmacokinetic mass was

100 to 108 kg, which illustrates the magnitude of dosing error that using TBW can lead to with fentanyl.

The situation with neuromuscular blockers is more consistent, which is not surprising given the polar, hydrophilic nature of nondepolarizing neuromuscular blockers, which tends to limit their volume of distribution. Vecuronium will have a prolonged duration of action if it is administered on the basis of TBW. If it is administered based on IBW, the volume of distribution, total clearance, and elimination half-life has been shown to be equivalent between obese and normal subjects [12]. A small study [13] comparing the effects of rocuronium dose based on TBW with effects based on IBW also concludes that rocuronium dosage in obese patients should be guided by IBW to avoid significant prolongation of the duration of action (55 min versus 22 min, until 25% twitch tension return). The same authors used a similar model to study the effects of cisatracurium in obese patients and found similar results, with dosage guided by TBW leading to a prolonged duration of action [14]. Thus, nondepolarizing neuromuscular blockers should be administered based on IBW to avoid prolonged duration of action.

Finally, in regard to volatile anesthetic gasses, which are commonly used in current clinical practice, two new drugs have become widely used over the past decade. Sevoflurane and desflurane offer lower blood solubility, which should speed anesthetic uptake, distribution, and also recovery from the anesthetic after drug delivery is terminated. Anesthetic vapors that are less likely to become widely distributed in fat and more likely to leave the body quickly after cessation of delivery should offer clinical advantages to morbidly obese patients.

Two studies [15,16] comparing the effects of isoflurane and sevoflurane in morbidly obese patients showed faster emergence after surgery with sevoflurane. A study [17] comparing sevoflurane and desflurane in obese patients showed faster emergence and marginally higher oxygen saturation in patients treated with desflurane. A third study [18] has compared recovery profiles after desflurane, isoflurane, and propofol and concludes that immediate and intermediate recovery are faster in patients who have received desflurane as the basis of their maintenance anesthetic.

Although the pharmacokinetic characteristics of the newer volatile anesthetic drugs offer the possibility of a more rapid emergence and faster immediate recovery, it is clear that all of the modern anesthetic vapors are safe to use in obese patients. If rapid initial emergence is of paramount importance, desflurane is the drug most likely to be chosen. Sevoflurane offers clinical advantages in certain situations (mask induction), and isoflurane offers a long record of safety and very low administration costs.

Positioning obese patients for surgery

There is no convincing body of literature that suggests that obese patients have more frequent complications from positioning during anesthesia than normal weight patients, but active clinicians know that standard techniques often do not work well in obese patients. Even the standard supine position may offer some difficulty because some patients are so big that standard operating room tables are either too small or are unable to handle the patient's weight. A recent report [19] describes rhabdomyolysis of the gluteal muscles leading to renal failure in several morbidly obese patients who were supine for 5-hour gastric bypass operations. Another case report [20] describes rhabdomyolysis leading to renal failure and death after bariatric surgery.

The prone position can be challenging because obese patients' bodies may not fit well into frames designed for normal weight individuals, and alternatives such as gel rolls are subject to excessive compression from the sheer weight placed on them. Pressure points must be carefully checked, and even then, skin breakdown can occur in cases of prolonged surgery. Proper planning is essential to minimize the risk of postoperative complications from pressure necrosis.

The lateral position offers its own challenges, with the downward hip subject to a substantial amount of pressure regardless of the type of padding placed under it. The patient's upward arm must be well padded and supported, and it may or may not be necessary to use a traditional axillary roll support, depending on the amount of soft tissue present under the patient.

The lithotomy position may be difficult because the weight of the patient's legs may exceed the capacity of the standard stirrups used to provide leg support in this position. Compartment syndrome has occurred as a complication of this position, and as with any other position, care must be taken when placing the patient in position, and every effort must be made to minimize the amount of time the patient spends in the lithotomy position [21].

As the obesity pandemic works its way through our society, health care organizations must plan appropriately for the care of morbidly obese patients and consider the safety of the health care workers involved in caring for these patients. Institutions with busy bariatric surgery programs should purchase special operating room tables and perhaps even motorized hospital beds to facilitate the transport of morbidly obese patients from the operating room to the recovery room and then to their hospital rooms. If it is necessary to move an anesthetized morbidly obese patient, either a roller should be used under the patient or enough personnel must be present to minimize the risk of injury to those moving the patient.

Regional anesthesia in obese patients

There is now extensive experience with regional anesthesia in morbidly obese patients from modern obstetric anesthetic practice. It is clear that spinal and epidural anesthesia are technically feasible and safe in this population of patients. It is also clear that it is technically more difficult, that indwelling catheters are more likely to migrate and that specially designed equipment may be necessary [22]. Continuous techniques such as continuous spinal anesthesia and spinal-epidural anesthesia have become more popular, especially when maternal cardiovascular disease makes a gradual onset of sympathetic block a desirable method [23,24]. With either spinal or epidural techniques, care should be taken in dosing, because obese patients are likely to have greater cephalad spread of sympathetic block than normal weight patients [25,26]. Obese patients will also experience greater respiratory embarrassment from a high regional block than normal weight patients will [27].

Whether postoperative epidural analgesia improves outcome remains controversial. The increasing use of laparoscopic techniques to replace procedures that previously required open laparotomy in obese patients has simplified the postoperative care required by many obese patients. In obese patients who require open laparotomy, vital capacity will decrease very significantly postoperatively. Thoracic epidural analgesia has been shown to reduce this decline in vital capacity and should be considered [28].

The continuing trend toward performing ambulatory surgical procedures ensures that many obese patients will present for ambulatory surgery. Many procedures can be performed under peripheral nerve block and sedation, or they can benefit from a peripheral nerve block to reduce postoperative pain. The development of continuous catheter techniques for postoperative pain relief offers the potential to significantly reduce postoperative pain. A recent report [29] on more than 9000 peripheral nerve blocks documents high patient satisfaction with peripheral nerve block in obese patients but also a higher rate of block failure and complications. The authors suggest that obese patients should not be excluded from consideration for peripheral nerve blocks in the ambulatory setting.

The intensity of monitoring required for obese patients

There is little evidence to suggest that the presence of obesity per se increases the intensity of monitoring required for the delivery of an anesthetic. Anesthesia for gastroplasty can be safely provided with or without invasive monitoring [30]. The presence of comorbidities, which will be more common among obese patients presenting for surgery, will lead to the more frequent use of invasive monitoring. Highly selected obese patients (such as those with obesity-hypoventilation syndrome who are likely to have pulmonary hypertension and cor pulmonale) may benefit from cardiovascular monitoring with a pulmonary artery catheter or transesophageal echocardiography and may require postoperative intensive care. Technical difficulty with peripheral venous access may lead to the need to insert central venous catheters to obtain adequate vascular access. If the insertion of a central venous catheter for vascular access proves to be necessary, strong consideration should be given to the use of ultrasonographic guidance, because the central catheter insertion may be technically difficult as well. It may be necessary to insert an arterial line to obtain reliable blood pressure readings in some morbidly obese individuals, because the body habitus may interfere with the performance of blood pressure cuffs.

Laparoscopy in obese patients

There is accumulating evidence to suggest that bariatric surgery offers continued reduction in comorbidities and the possibility of long-term weight reduction to obese patients [2]. The widespread introduction of laparoscopic gastric bypass has led to extensive experience with laparoscopy in morbidly obese individuals. Laparoscopy requires intra-abdominal insufflation of a gas, usually carbon dioxide, to provide a pneumoperitoneum that allows visualization of and access to intra-abdominal structures. The creation of a pneumoperitoneum increases intra-abdominal pressure (IAP), which has cardiovascular consequences that vary with the level of intra-abdominal pressure. Systemic vascular resistance increases with the creation of pneumoperitoneum, and low levels of IAP (≥ 10 mm Hg) increase venous return, with a resultant increase in arterial blood pressure and cardiac output. Higher levels of IAP can obstruct the vena cava, leading to decreased venous return and hence decreased cardiac output [31].

Increased intra-abdominal pressure can reduce urine output, but experience with laparoscopic kidney donation documents that a management strategy designed to avoid hypovolemia and preserve renal perfusion pressure results in excellent renal function in both the donated and remaining kidneys [32]. In the absence of hemorrhage and with intra-abdominal pressure limited to 12 to 15 mm Hg, it does not appear to be necessary to administer additional fluid (in excess of that required to replace the preoperative fluid deficit, plus intraoperative maintenance and blood loss) to ensure preservation of renal function.

Respiratory mechanics are impaired by both severe obesity and by the creation of pneumoperitoneum. Functional residual capacity is reduced in obesity, and atelectasis can be a significant clinical problem in the perioperative period [33]. Decreased pulmonary compliance has been documented in obese patients undergoing laparoscopy, and pneumoperitoneum worsens compliance and leads to increased requirements for CO_2 elimination, which will require increases in ventilation. Anesthetized morbidly obese patients in the supine position had 29% lower pulmonary compliance than normal weight patients in one study [34], and unfortunately neither a doubling of tidal volume nor a doubling of respiratory frequency reduced the alveolar-arterial gradient. The endotracheal tube position must be carefully monitored in obese patients undergoing laparoscopy, because the head-downward position and abdominal insufflation can cause migration of the endotracheal tube into the right mainstem bronchus [35]. Despite these problems, laparoscopy is usually well tolerated as long as the pneumoperitoneum pressure is maintained at less than 15 mm Hg, and many studies [36] show reductions in overall morbidity when a laparoscopic technique is used.

Minimizing hypoxia during anesthesia

It has been recognized for many years that obese individuals are more likely to become hypoxic during anesthesia and surgery than normal weight patients [37] are. Obese patients desaturate more quickly when apnea is caused by general anesthesia, which makes careful preoxygenation extremely important [38]. Morbid obesity is associated with reductions in expiratory reserve volume, forced vital capacity, forced expiratory volume $(FEV)_1$, functional residual capacity (FRC), and maximum voluntary ventilation [39]. Marked derangements in lung and chest wall mechanics have been well documented in mechanically ventilated and paralyzed morbidly obese patients, including reduced respiratory system compliance, increased respiratory system resistance, severely reduced FRC, and impaired arterial oxygenation [40]. BMI is an important determinant of lung volumes, respiratory mechanics, and oxygenation, with increasing BMI leading to exponential decreases in FRC, total lung compliance, and oxygenation index (partial pressure $[PAO_2]/PAO_2$), whereas chest wall compliance was only minimally affected [41]. Hypoxemia during mechanical ventilation in obese patients is mediated at least in part through unopposed increases in intra-abdominal pressure that reduce lung volumes, resulting in ventilation-perfusion mismatch [42].

The myriad respiratory dysfunctions described above make it important to take advantage of techniques that can reduce the degree of intraoperative hypoxemia that occurs in obese patients. Induction of anesthesia in obese patients must be performed in a cautious manner. If careful preoperative evaluation raises any question about the adequacy of the mask airway, an awake intubation technique should be considered. The proper positioning for direct laryngoscopy will maximize the likelihood of success on the first attempt, and it may require significant elevation of the upper body and head [43]. Positioning obese patients in a "ramped" position (with blankets used to elevate both the upper body and head of the patient) has been shown to result in improved laryngeal exposure with direct laryngoscopy, which should result in fewer failed intubations [44]. The difficulty of repositioning a morbidly obese patient during a failed intubation should not be underestimated, and proper positioning is often not understood or perceived by practitioners who are not experienced in airway management in obese patients. If direct laryngoscopy is unsuccessful, laryngeal mask airways are effective for establishing ventilation and should be immediately available [45].

The prevention or reduction of atelectasis from the induction and maintenance of general anesthesia would improve arterial oxygenation. Preoxygenation with 100% fraction of inspired oxygen (FIO_2) and 10-cm positive end-expiratory pressure (PEEP) for 5 minutes before the induction of general anesthesia followed by 10-cm PEEP during mask ventilation and after intubation reduces immediate postintubation atelectasis as assessed by CT scan and improves immediate post-intubation arterial oxygenation on 100% FIO_2 (PAO_2 of 457 $\pm$ 130 mm Hg versus 315 $\pm$ 100 mm Hg in the control group) [46]. Whether this reduction is maintained and for how long it is maintained are not known. The application of 10 cm of PEEP during the maintenance phase of general anesthesia has been shown to provide a sustained improvement in arterial oxygenation in morbidly obese patients through alveolar recruitment [47]. Although these maneuvers are safe in most patients, further clinical studies with PEEP in obese patients would be helpful, particularly concerning the application of PEEP during induction. Whether PEEP is safe and effective during induction in patients with gastroesophageal reflux and an incompetent gastroesophageal junction has not yet been determined. In obese patients without reflux, the improvement in oxygenation that can be achieved with the preinduction use of PEEP is significant and will increase the time period before desaturation begins. Practitioners should strongly consider taking advantage of the improved arterial oxygenation that preinduction PEEP offers.

Anesthetic management of patients with sleep apnea

Sleep apnea is a general term for several conditions that involve sleep-disordered breathing. The most common type of sleep apnea is obstructive sleep apnea (OSA), which involves obstruction of the airway during sleep (for airway management and preoperative and postoperative management, see discussion elsewhere in this issue). The anesthetic care of patients with OSA is challenging because anesthetic drugs profoundly influence control of the respiratory system, which is already dysfunctional, and because many patients with OSA have significant comorbidities [48,49]. This section will discuss the effects of anesthetic drugs on ventilatory responses to hypercarbia and hypoxemia, the lack of evidence for the superiority of a specific anesthetic technique, the intensity of monitoring required, and rational, if not evidence-based, strategies to minimize perioperative morbidity in patients with OSA.

Many questions central to the anesthetic management of patients with OSA have not been addressed by well-done clinical trials. Whether perioperative risk is altered by anesthetic technique (ie, inhalational general, intravenous general, regional anesthesia, or local anesthesia with sedation) is not known. For non-airway surgery in patients with OSA, little information exists on which to base decisions regarding the appropriate postoperative setting and the degree of special, if any, postoperative monitoring is required by these patients. The literature does not provide evidence-based guidance regarding whether patients with OSA can safely undergo outpatient surgery or whether all patients with OSA require hospital monitoring after their surgery.

The effect of anesthetic drugs on ventilatory responses in patients with obstructive sleep apnea

There is evidence that many anesthetic agents cause exaggerated responses in patients with sleep apnea. Drugs such as pentothal, propofol, opioids, benzodiazepines, and nitrous oxide may reduce the tone of the pharyngeal musculature that acts to maintain airway patency [50,51]. The response to carbon dioxide in children with OSA and tonsillar hypertrophy is diminished during halothane anesthesia [52]. Intubated, spontaneously breathing children with sleep apnea who are anesthetized with a volatile anesthetic have depressed ventilation compared with normal children and an incidence of up to 50% apnea after 0.5 μg/kg of fentanyl is administered [53]. Although the studies cited above regarding ventilatory response to carbon dioxide and apnea after modest doses of fentanyl were performed in children, prudence dictates that these conditions be considered when formulating anesthetic plans for adult patients with OSA. Studies such as these, and common sense, make it reasonable to assume that sleep apnea will be worsened postoperatively. Anesthesia techniques using shorter-acting drugs are attractive because it would be reasonable to expect a more rapid return to baseline respiratory function when shorter-acting drugs are used.

Anesthesia technique

Unfortunately, no evidence exists regarding whether perioperative risk in patients with sleep apnea depends on the type of anesthetic technique employed. The available information suggests it is the type of surgery (eg, minor versus major or invasive surgery) that makes a difference in outcome. Anesthesia techniques, including regional anesthesia, that minimize the use of sedatives in an effort to minimize respiratory depression or allow a rapid restoration of consciousness after emergence from general anesthesia may be desirable in specific clinical situations. Regional anesthesia does offer the possibility of minimally affecting respiratory drive and can reduce the affect of anesthetic agents on subsequent sleep patterns as well as maintain arousal responses during apneic episodes. Sedation must be carefully administered and monitored, because sedatives will worsen hypoventilation in patients with sleep apnea [54,55].

Intensity of intraoperative monitoring required

There is no evidence to suggest that patients with OSA need more aggressive, intensive, or invasive intraoperative monitoring than normal patients do. The intensity of monitoring should be dictated by the type of surgery planned and by other comorbidities the patient brings to the operating room. Transesophageal echocardiography is often used as a monitor of ventricular filling and function for noncardiac surgery, but it will not be useful for any surgery involving the airway. If the patient with sleep apnea is morbidly obese, an intra-arterial catheter may be necessary if noninvasive blood pressure monitoring is unreliable or not possible for technical reasons. Metabolic alkalosis can result in mild hypoventilation, which is undesirable in these patients. Thus, the maintenance of the patient's baseline bicarbonate is appropriate.

A rational approach to guide anesthetic management in patients with obstructive sleep apnea

Regardless of the type of anesthetic planned, the management of the airway should be conservative, with measures taken to minimize hypoxia secondary to airway obstruction or apnea. Patients should be monitored and observed if sedation is administered, and sedative drugs should be administered in a cautious, titrated fashion. If spontaneous ventilation is to be ablated, strict attention to adequate preoxygenation is mandatory, and laryngeal mask airways and other emergency airway devices should be immediately available. Regional anesthesia can be used in many situations, but heavy sedation in conjunction with regional anesthesia may be problematic in this patient group because of airway obstruction. The pharyngeal cross-sectional area is larger in the lateral position than in the supine position, which may limit airway obstruction in procedures performed under regional anesthesia in the lateral position [56].

The maintenance of general anesthesia can be managed with volatile anesthetic vapors or intravenous anesthetics, but strong consideration should be given to the use of newer, shorter-acting drugs to minimize the duration of postoperative ventilatory depression. Extubation should be accomplished as with other patients. If the patient had a difficult airway, extubation should be accomplished in a conservative fashion. There should be an assessment of the patient's strength and level of consciousness. Careful antagonism of neuromuscular blockade should be accomplished, and the effectiveness of antagonism should be carefully assessed, as should the possibility of residual levels of fixed or inhalational agents.

The provision of adequate postoperative analgesia is an integral part of the anesthetic plan, and it should be accomplished, to the extent possible, in a multimodal fashion. Sedation and narcotic-based analgesia may exacerbate symptoms of sleep apnea. However, there are no adequately powered studies to guide analgesic therapy of these patients. There are case reports [57,58] of adverse respiratory events occurring with analgesia administered through both the parenteral and epidural routes, including patient-controlled analgesia. The use of nonsteroidal anti-inflammatory drugs, local anesthetics for incision infiltration, and epidural analgesia and peripheral nerve blocks, when appropriate, can minimize the necessity for the administration of large doses of narcotic drugs to achieve adequate analgesia. Regional analgesic techniques may be helpful in postoperative management of these patients, although whether these techniques reduce the incidence of sleep-disordered breathing postoperatively is unknown.

References

[1] Hedley AA, Ogden CL, Carroll MD, et al. Prevalence of overweight and obesity among US children, adolescents, and adults, 1999–2002. JAMA 2004;291:2847–50.

[2] Sjostrom L, Lindroos AK, Peltonen M, et al. Lifestyle, diabetes, and cardiovascular risk factors 10 years after bariatric surgery. N Engl J Med 2004;351(26):2683–93.

[3] Christou NV, Sampalis JS, Liberman M, et al. Surgery decreases long-term mortality, morbidity, and health care use in morbidly obese patients. Ann Surg 2004;240(3):416–23.

[4] Cheymol G. Effects of obesity on pharmacokinetics implications for drug therapy. Clin Pharmacokinet 2000;39(3):215–31.

[5] Rowland M, Tozer TN. Distribution. In: Rowland M, Tozer TN, editors. Clinical pharmacokinetics: concepts and applications. 3rd edition. Baltimore: Williams & Wilkins; 1995. p. 137–55.

[6] Reisin E, Tuck ML. Obesity-associated hypertension: hypothesized link between etiology and selection of therapy. Blood Press Monit 1999;4(Suppl 1):S23–6.

[7] Messerli FH, Christie B, DeCarvalho JG, et al. Obesity and essential hypertension. Hemodynamics, intravascular volume, sodium excretion, and plasma renin activity. Arch Intern Med 1981;141(1):81–5.

[8] Servin F, Farinotti R, Haberer JP, et al. Propofol infusion for maintenance of anesthesia in morbidly obese patients receiving nitrous oxide: a clinical and pharmacokinetic study. Anesthesiology 1993;78(4):657–65.

[9] Egan TD, Hulzinga B, Gupta SK, et al. Remifentanil pharmacokinetics in obese versus lean patients. Anesthesiology 1998;89(3):562–73.

[10] Slepchenko G, Simon N, Goubaux B, et al. Performance of target-controlled sufentanil infusion in obese patients. Anesthesiology 2003;98(1):65–73.

[11] Shibutani K, Inchiosa MA, Sawada K, et al. Accuracy of pharmacokinetic models for predicting plasma fentanyl concentrations in lean and obese surgical patients: derivation of dosing weight ("pharmacokinetic mass"). Anesthesiology 2004;101(3):603–13.

[12] Schwartz AE, Matteo RS, Ornstein E, et al. Pharmacokinetics and pharmacodynamics of vecuronium in the obese surgical patient. Anesth Analg 1992;74(4):515–8.

[13] Leykin Y, Pellis T, Lucca M, et al. The pharmacodynamic effects of rocuronium when dosed according to real body weight or ideal body weight in morbidly obese patients. Anesth Analg 2004;99(4):1086–9 [table of contents].

[14] Leykin Y, Pellis T, Lucca M, et al. The effects of cisatracurium on morbidly obese women. Anesth Analg 2004;99(4):1090–4 [table of contents].

[15] Torri G, Casati A, Albertin A, et al. Randomized comparison of isoflurane and sevoflurane for laparoscopic gastric banding in morbidly obese patients. J Clin Anesth 2001;13(8):565–70.

[16] Sollazzi L, Perilli V, Modesti C, et al. Volatile anesthesia in bariatric surgery. Obes Surg 2001; 11(5):623–6.

[17] Strum EM, Szenohradszki J, Kaufman WA, et al. Emergence and recovery characteristics of desflurane versus sevoflurane in morbidly obese adult surgical patients: a prospective, randomized study. Anesth Analg 2004;99(6):1848–53 [table of contents].

[18] Juvin P, Vadam C, Malek L, et al. Postoperative recovery after desflurane, propofol, or isoflurane anesthesia among morbidly obese patients: a prospective, randomized study. Anesth Analg 2000; 91(3):714–9.

[19] Bostanjian D, Anthone GJ, Hamouti N, et al. Rhabdomyolysis of gluteal muscles leading to renal failure: a potentially fatal complication of surgery in the morbidly obese. Obes Surg 2003;13(2): 302–5.

[20] Collier B, Goreja MA, Duke III BE. Postoperative rhabdomyolysis with bariatric surgery. Obes Surg 2003;13(6):941–3.

[21] Mathews PV, Perry JJ, Murray PC. Compartment syndrome of the well leg as a result of the hemilithotomy position: a report of two cases and review of literature. J Orthop Trauma 2001; 15(8):580–3.

[22] Hood DD, Dewan DM. Anesthetic and obstetric outcome in morbidly obese parturients. Anesthesiology 1993;79(6):1210–8.

[23] Shnaider R, Ezri T, Szmuk P, et al. Combined spinal-epidural anesthesia for Cesarean section in a patient with peripartum dilated cardiomyopathy. Can J Anaesth 2001;48(7):681–3.

[24] Coker LL. Continuous spinal anesthesia for cesarean section for a morbidly obese parturient patient: a case report. J Am Assoc Nurse Anesth 2002;70(3):189–92.

[25] Hodgkinson R, Husain FJ. Obesity and the cephalad spread of analgesia following epidural administration of bupivacaine for Cesarean section. Anesth Analg 1980;59(2):89–92.
[26] Hodgkinson R, Husain FJ. Obesity, gravity, and spread of epidural anesthesia. Anesth Analg 1981;60(6):421–4.
[27] von Ungern-Sternberg BS, Regli A, Bucher E, et al. Impact of spinal anaesthesia and obesity on maternal respiratory function during elective Caesarean section. Anaesthesia 2004;59(8):743–9.
[28] von Ungern-Sternberg BS, Regli A, Reber A, et al. Effect of obesity and thoracic epidural analgesia on perioperative spirometry. Br J Anaesth 2005;94(1):121–7.
[29] Nielsen KC, Guller U, Steele SM, et al. Influence of obesity on surgical regional anesthesia in the ambulatory setting: an analysis of 9,038 blocks. Anesthesiology 2005;102(1):181–7.
[30] Capella JF, Capella RF. Is routine invasive monitoring indicated in surgery for the morbidly obese? Obes Surg 1996;6(1):50–3.
[31] Ogunnaike BO, Jones SB, Jones DB, et al. Anesthetic considerations for bariatric surgery. Anesth Analg 2002;95(6):1793–805.
[32] Biancofiore G, Amorose G, Lugli D, et al. Perioperative anesthetic management for laparoscopic kidney donation. Transplant Proc 2004;36(3):464–6.
[33] Eichenberger A, Proietti S, Wicky S, et al. Morbid obesity and postoperative pulmonary atelectasis: an underestimated problem. Anesth Analg 2002;95(6):1788–92 [table of contents].
[34] Sprung J, Whalley DG, Falcone T, et al. The effects of tidal volume and respiratory rate on oxygenation and respiratory mechanics during laparoscopy in morbidly obese patients. Anesth Analg 2003;97(1):268–74 [table of contents].
[35] Ezri T, Hazin V, Warters D, et al. The endotracheal tube moves more often in obese patients undergoing laparoscopy compared with open abdominal surgery. Anesth Analg 2003;96(1):278–82 [table of contents].
[36] Lamvu G, Zolnoun D, Boggess J, et al. Obesity: physiologic changes and challenges during laparoscopy. Am J Obstet Gynecol 2004;191(2):669–74.
[37] Vaughan RW, Wise L. Intraoperative arterial oxygenation in obese patients. Ann Surg 1976;184(1):35–42.
[38] Jense HG, Dubin SA, Silverstein PL, et al. Effect of obesity on safe duration of apnea in anesthetized humans. Anesth Analg 1991;72(1):89–93.
[39] Biring MS, Lewis MI, Liu JT, et al. Pulmonary physiologic changes of morbid obesity. Am J Med Sci 1999;318(5):293–7.
[40] Pelosi P, Croci M, Ravagnan I, et al. Total respiratory system, lung, and chest wall mechanics in sedated-paralyzed postoperative morbidly obese patients. Chest 1996;109(1):144–51.
[41] Pelosi P, Croci M, Ravagnan I, et al. The effects of body mass on lung volumes, respiratory mechanics, and gas exchange during general anesthesia. Anesth Analg 1998;87(3):654–60.
[42] Pelosi P, Croci M, Ravagnan I, et al. Respiratory system mechanics in sedated, paralyzed, morbidly obese patients. J Appl Physiol 1997;82(3):811–8.
[43] Brodsky JB, Lemmens HJ, Brock-Utne JG, et al. Anesthetic considerations for bariatric surgery: proper positioning is important for laryngoscopy. Anesth Analg 2003;96(6):1841–2 [author reply, 1842].
[44] Collins JS, Lemmens HJ, Brodsky JB, et al. Laryngoscopy and morbid obesity: a comparison of the "sniff" and "ramped" positions. Obes Surg 2004;14(9):1171–5.
[45] Frappier J, Guenon T, Journois D, et al. Airway management using the intubating laryngeal mask airway for the morbidly obese patient. Anesth Analg 2003;96(5):1510–5 [table of contents].
[46] Coussa M, Proietti S, Schnyder P, et al. Prevention of atelectasis formation during the induction of general anesthesia in morbidly obese patients. Anesth Analg 2004;98(5):1491–5 [table of contents].
[47] Pelosi P, Ravagnan I, Giurati G, et al. Positive end-expiratory pressure improves respiratory function in obese but not in normal subjects during anesthesia and paralysis. Anesthesiology 1999;91(5):1221–31.
[48] Hillman DR, Loadsman JA, Platt PR, et al. Obstructive sleep apnoea and anaesthesia. Sleep Med Rev 2004;8(6):459–71.

[49] Loadsman JA, Hillman DR. Anaesthesia and sleep apnoea. Br J Anaesth 2001;86(2):254–66.
[50] Dhonneur G, Combes X, Leroux B, et al. Postoperative obstructive apnea. Anesth Analg 1999; 89(3):762–7.
[51] Benumof JL. Obstructive sleep apnea in the adult obese patient: implications for airway management. J Clin Anesth 2001;13(2):144–56.
[52] Strauss SG, Lynn AM, Bratton SL, et al. Ventilatory response to CO2 in children with obstructive sleep apnea from adenotonsillar hypertrophy. Anesth Analg 1999;89(2):328–32.
[53] Waters KA, McBrien F, Stewart P, et al. Effects of OSA, inhalational anesthesia, and fentanyl on the airway and ventilation of children. J Appl Physiol 2002;92(5):1987–94.
[54] Catley DM, Thornton C, Jordan C, et al. Pronounced, episodic oxygen desaturation in the postoperative period: its association with ventilatory pattern and analgesic regimen. Anesthesiology 1985;63(1):20–8.
[55] Dolly FR, Block AJ. Effect of flurazepam on sleep-disordered breathing and nocturnal oxygen desaturation in asymptomatic subjects. Am J Med 1982;73(2):239–43.
[56] Isono S, Tanaka A, Nishino T. Lateral position decreases collapsibility of the passive pharynx in patients with obstructive sleep apnea. Anesthesiology 2002;97(4):780–5.
[57] Stone JG, Cozine KA, Wald A. Nocturnal oxygenation during patient-controlled analgesia. Anesth Analg 1999;89(1):104–10.
[58] VanDercar DH, Martinez AP, De Lisser EA. Sleep apnea syndromes: a potential contraindication for patient-controlled analgesia. Anesthesiology 1991;74(3):623–4.

ELSEVIER
SAUNDERS

Anesthesiology Clin N Am
23 (2005) 493–500

ANESTHESIOLOGY
CLINICS OF
NORTH AMERICA

Postoperative Considerations for Patients with Obesity and Sleep Apnea

Robert L. Bell, MD, MA[a,*], Stanley H. Rosenbaum, MD[b,c]

[a]Department of Surgery, Yale University School of Medicine, 40 Temple Street, Suite 3A,
New Haven, CT 06510, USA
[b]Department of Anesthesiology, Yale University School of Medicine, 333 Cedar Street, TMP 3,
P.O. Box 208051, New Haven, CT 06520-8051, USA
[c]Private practice, 333 Cedar Street, TMP 3, P.O. Box 208051, New Haven, CT 06520-8051, USA

Over the past several decades, obesity has developed into a series health problem of epidemic proportions. Few countries have escaped this phenomenon, but obesity is most prevalent in the Unites States. Obesity is most commonly defined using the body mass index (BMI) criterion. BMI is expressed as a ratio of weight (kg) to height (m^2). Normal BMI range from 19.5 to 24.9 kg/m^2, overweight is defined as a range of 25.0 to 29.9 kg/m^2, and obesity is defined by a BMI greater than 30 kg/m^2. Current estimates are that 65% of US adults are classified as overweight or obese, over 30% of adults are classified as obese, and the prevalence of obesity has doubled over the past 20 years [1]. Accounting for over 400,000 deaths annually, obesity is second only to tobacco-related disease as a cause of preventable and premature death [2]. With the increasing obesity health epidemic, an increase in obesity-related health problems also has been seen. The prevalence of diabetes has increased by 33% over the past 10 years [3], and the prevalence of hypertension has doubled over the past 25 years, from 15% in 1976 to 30.1% in 2000 [4,5].

* Corresponding author.
  E-mail address: robert.bell@yale.edu (R.L. Bell).

0889-8537/05/$ – see front matter © 2005 Elsevier Inc. All rights reserved.
doi:10.1016/j.atc.2005.03.007
anesthesiology.theclinics.com

Epidemiology of obstructive sleep apnea

Obstructive sleep apnea (OSA), a well-recognized comorbid illness of obesity, is a relatively new disease in its strictest definition. Charles Dickens' famous novel of 1837, *The Posthumous Papers of the Pickwick Club*, describes a character named Joe who is obese and always sleepy. Sir William Osler [6] later described any obese and sleepy person as "Pickwickian." This eloquent but medically nondescript term has persisted until recently. It was not until the field of sleep medicine was established in the 1960s and 1970s that such Pickwickian patients' sleep patterns were examined and the sleep apnea syndromes were more precisely defined [7,8].

The prevalence of OSA depends on the methodology of defining patients with sleep apnea, but the prevalence of OSA is estimated to be 4% in men and 2% in women [9]. OSA is a serious, life-threatening condition with an estimated 8-year mortality rate of nearly 40% [10]. Obesity is a well-established risk factor for sleep apnea, with the incidence of OSA increasing in direct proportion with the level of obesity [11–13]. For patients with clinically severe obesity (BMI ≥ 35 kg/m^2) who present for bariatric surgery, the incidence of sleep apnea ranges from 71% to 77% [14,15]. In addition to obesity, other comorbidities associated with OSA include hypertension, stroke, congestive heart failure, coronary artery disease, cardiac arrhythmias, and pulmonary hypertension [16]. Although the precise mechanisms of these comorbid conditions are incompletely understood, they most likely result from a combination of chronic hypoxemia, chronic hypercarbia, and hemodynamic changes associated with the inappropriate termination of sleep.

Pathophysiology of sleep apnea

The sine qua non of obstructive sleep apnea is the physical collapse of the pharyngeal airway during sleep. This phenomenon should be distinguished from central sleep apnea, which results from the physiologic inhibition of breathing. In obstructive sleep apnea, the upper pharyngeal muscles lose tone during sleep, which leads to a narrowing of the upper-airway. Problems stem from an individual's progressive attempts to inhale against a partially occluded airway. The phenomenon of OSA is compounded in obese individuals, from both a physical and physiologic standpoint. The weight and distribution of soft tissue fatty infiltration in patients with larger necks leads to turbulent airflow within the upper pharynx. The shear weight of such structures also tends to collapse the upper-airway musculature resulting from direct compression [17]. The culmination of these physical impediments leads to intermittent reduction of the alveolar oxygen saturation. Additionally, obese individuals exhibit a decrease in expiratory reserve volume and a reduction in all lung volumes. As an individual becomes more obese, the muscular work required and concomitant total body oxygen consumption increases. In patients with OSA, this places further demands on an already diminished alveolar oxygen saturation [18].

Implications during recovery and the immediate postoperative period

The intraoperative anesthetic management of patients with OSA merits special attention and has been reviewed by Boushra [19]. See the article by Passannante and Rock elsewhere in this issue for further exploration of this topic. Postoperatively, these patients present an additional challenge, beginning with their stay in the postanesthesia care unit (PACU). While they are in the PACU, all patients are continually monitored and frequently assessed for signs and symptoms of airway problems. Of all the patients admitted to the PACU, approximately 1 in 500 patients will require reintubation [20]. Obese patients and patients with OSA deserve special attention because they may be very difficult to intubate. In a recent study by Siyam and Benhamou [21], difficult intubation occurred in 21.9% of patients with OSA, compared with 2.6% in control subjects. Furthermore, in obese patients, neck circumference not BMI is predictive of difficult intubation [22].

Pharmacologic sedation has been shown to decrease upper pharyngeal muscle tone. Although decreased muscle tone is well tolerated in most patients, the combination of OSA and sedation could lead to airway compromise. Continuous oxygen should be provided through a nasal cannula or facemask to maintain adequate arterial oxygen saturation. Continuous positive airway pressure (CPAP), which may be delivered through a nasal or oronasal facemask, may also be necessary in patients who exhibit signs of upper-airway collapse while they are in the recovery room. For patients who arrive at the recovery room with a nasogastric tube in place, the nasal CPAP mask will not likely provide an adequate seal, making its use impractical in this subset of patients.

Particular attention to posture and positioning are very important in patients with OSA. The head of the patient's bed (HOB) should be elevated to at least 30°. Upper body elevation relieves OSA by increasing the stability of the upper airway [23]. The HOB position to 30° should be used by the OSA patient at all times while in the PACU and throughout his or her hospital stay.

Adequate blood pressure control should be the next focus of care for the OSA patient while in the recovery room. Postoperative hypertension may result from pain, hypercarbia, or anxiety. Of those patients who experience acute postoperative hypertension, almost 60% have a history of hypertension [24]. Given the high incidence of pre-existing hypertension in obese patients with OSA, invasive arterial monitoring should be considered while the patient is under general anesthesia, especially because standard, oscillometric, blood pressure cuffs have proven unreliable. Newer, noninvasive blood pressure monitors, such as the Vasotrac device (Medwave, Arden Hills, MN), also may prove useful in obese individuals [25]. The Vasotrac, placed around the wrist of the patient, continuously measures pulse and blood pressure and will provide an arterial waveform similar to that of an invasive arterial line. Such a device, if used during the operative procedure, would also prove useful while the patient is in the PACU.

Disposition from the postanesthesia care unit

Once the patient has recovered adequately from surgery, preparations need to be made to transfer the patient to the home, a standard medical or surgical unit, or an ICU. This is perhaps the most difficult category of decision-making for managing the patient with morbid obesity and OSA. In the setting of OSA, it is important to know the patient's preoperative apnea-hypopnea index and his or her dependence on CPAP for sleep, both of which yield valuable information about the vulnerability of the patient's airway. Other factors to be considered in determining postoperative placement include the presence of right or left ventricular heart failure, the presence of underlying lung disease, the degree of obesity, and the nature of the surgery. Patients with mild sleep apnea and minimal comorbidities who have undergone minor surgical procedures will likely be discharged home on the day of surgery. For patients with moderate sleep apnea and intermediate comorbidities who have undergone intermediate-risk surgery, admission to a standard medical or surgical unit should suffice. Patients with severe sleep apnea who require home CPAP or those with numerous comorbidities merit closer observation in an intermediate care unit or an intensive care unit, depending on the nature of the surgical procedure. The most suitable postoperative environment is also determined by the particular conditions within each hospital. There is scant sense in placing a patient on a ward nursing unit with oximetric monitoring if the nursing coverage at night is too thin for the alarms to be noted.

Fortunately, most complications that require more intensive postoperative observation become manifest in the recovery room within the first 2 hours of surgery [26]. More intensive monitoring also may be required depending on the presence or absence of intraoperative complications.

Some of the specific postoperative risks go beyond the simple presence of OSA. It is not uncommon for patients with OSA to have congestive heart failure, right- or left-sided, resulting from either systolic or diastolic dysfunction [16]. In that setting, postoperative fluid shifts will be more difficult to manage than in the typical patient. Aggressive postoperative fluid administration may lead to or worsen biventricular heart failure. Furthermore, in the setting of severe peripheral edema, fluid mobilization from the legs can occur when placing the patient from a long-term sitting position to the supine position, leading to cardiac decompensation from acute volume overload.

The importance of adequate blood pressure control in the immediate postoperative period cannot be overstated. As mentioned previously, patients with OSA have a high incidence of hypertension. Unfortunately, postoperative hypertension, which might result from pain or anxiety, could result in surgical site bleeding. In patients with OSA, narcotics and sedatives should be used judiciously and perioperative α- and β-blockade may need to be used. Therefore, patients with OSA and postoperative hypertension deserve closer postoperative monitoring.

Postoperative pain management

Patients do and should expect adequate pain relief following surgery. When properly administered, narcotic analgesics provide safe and effective control of postoperative pain. Postoperatively, patients with OSA present the anesthesiologist, surgeon, and nursing staff with a difficult situation. Although diminution of pain is the goal of every caregiver, the use of narcotics is especially dangerous in patients with OSA. After the use of any general anesthetic, the patient with OSA will exhibit a propensity for rapid eye movement (REM) sleep during the first several days after surgery [27]. In the patient with OSA, the genioglossus muscle is virtually paralyzed during REM sleep, allowing the tongue to fall posteriorly to the retroglossal space [28]. Normally, such patients would arouse and terminate REM sleep, but this reflex is diminished with the administration of narcotics or sedatives. For patients with severe pain and the need for opiates, the risk of over-sedation and airway compromise is clearly increased. Because it is reasonable to be concerned that the OSA will be worsened in the postoperative period, an assessment of the patient's baseline respiratory difficulty may aid in determining the postoperative vulnerability.

In patients with OSA, respiratory depression culminating in respiratory arrest has been reported after an intravenous "push" of opioid analgesics [29], an epidural infusion of opioid analgesia [30,31], and with the use of patient-controlled opioid analgesia [32]. Such respiratory events can be prevented with proper patient positioning (eg, HOB to 30°), the administration of CPAP, and the limited use of narcotic analgesics. Nonsteroidal anti-inflammatory drugs (NSAIDs) should be used as an adjunct for postoperative pain control. Ostermeier et al [31] have noted that the use of NSAIDs can decrease opioid use by 20% to 35%.

The first line of therapy whenever respiratory depression occurs includes the provision of supplemental oxygen and the careful titration of intravenous naloxone. If this approach fails, a nasal or oral airway may immediately temporize the problem, and CPAP should be administered as soon as possible. Positioning the patient in a sitting position also may be beneficial.

Patients whose respiratory depression fails to respond to the aforementioned measures or any patient in respiratory failure will need emergency endotracheal intubation. Endotracheal intubation may be difficult in such patients, as would emergency cricothyroidotomy. The very obese patient can desaturate very rapidly, and cardiac arrest can occur surprisingly fast. Skilled airway management is crucial. Even if the patient is known from recent operating room experience to be an "easy intubation," the potential difficulty in the emergency setting must be appreciated. The hard operating room table, where the patient is in a perfect intubating position, is very different from the soft hospital bed, with a large, strong, struggling patient. In the awake and breathing patient, the intubation may need to be performed with the patient sitting up, either through a "blind" nasal technique or with the use of a fiber-optic bronchoscope, also often performed though the nasal route.

Additional considerations for the obese patient

Ambulation of the severely obese patient (BMI ≥ 60 kg/m^2), many of whom will have degenerative joint disease, presents a special challenge. In the setting of postoperative pain or sedation, early ambulation and even proper postural positioning while in bed, although crucial, may prove to be very difficult. Many obese patients prefer to sleep sitting up, and in such patients, respiration is very uncomfortable in the flat, supine position. Respiration will be compromised ultimately if pain, weakness, or inadequate labor constrains the patient to a supine position. The nursing staff needs to be educated about the importance of proper positioning and early mobility. Assisting these very large patients with ambulation may easily overwhelm a typical medical-surgical floor nursing staff. Therefore, physical therapy should be generously prescribed to ensure appropriate ambulation after surgery.

Skin breakdown is another special concern in the obese patient in the postoperative setting. Adequate oxygen delivery to the skin and subcutaneous tissue is determined foremost by cardiac function, specifically cardiac output, and by respiratory function, which establishes the level of hemoglobin saturation and the partial pressure of arterial oxygen. As mentioned previously, both cardiac and respiratory function may be impaired, especially in the setting of OSA. The impairment is compounded by the poor vascularity of adipose tissue, which further predisposes to soft tissue ischemia. Pressure sores are likely to develop in these individuals if they are not appropriately padded, turned, and repositioned [33]. Unfortunately, obese individuals may be difficult to reposition, often requiring several staff members to adequately turn the patient. Excessive adipose tissue should not be viewed as extra padding. Rather, proper padding of the upper and lower extremities is essential. Until the patient ambulates freely, padding should be placed underneath the patient's calves to avoid any pressure on the heels. This point further emphasizes the need for appropriate nursing education to avoid these otherwise avoidable complications.

Summary

Sleep apnea and obesity are two prevalent and often coexisting conditions that are a challenge to treat medically, anesthetically, and surgically. Any obese patient with OSA who undergoes surgery requires a thorough preoperative evaluation. A knowledge of the magnitude of the sleep disorder as well as concomitant medical comorbidities leads to the proper appraisal of anesthetic and operative risks. Although routine monitoring in the ICU is unnecessary, high-risk patients should be monitored postoperatively in an ICU-type setting. Realizing that the overzealous use of opioids in patients with OSA can lead to respiratory arrest, pain control should include the use of NSAIDs to help minimize the use of narcotics.

References

[1] Flegal KM, Carroll MD, Ogden CL, et al. Prevalence and trends in obesity among US adults, 1999–2000. JAMA 2002;288(14):1723–7.

[2] World Health Organization. Obesity: preventing and managing the global epidemic: report of a WHO consultation. World Health Organ Tech Rep Ser 2000;894:1–253.

[3] Caprio S. Obesity and type 2 diabetes: the twin epidemic. Diabetes Spectrum 2003;4:230.

[4] Labarthe DR. The prevalence of hypertension in the United States today. Drugs 1976;11(Suppl 1): S11–5.

[5] National Center for Health Statistics. Available at: http://www.cdc.gov/nchs/fastats/hyprtens.htm. Accessed April 18, 2005.

[6] Osler W. The principles and practice of medicine. New York: Appleton; 1906. p. 431.

[7] Gastaut H, Tassinari CA, Duran B, et al. Polygraphic study of episodic diurnal and nocturnal manifestations of the Pickwickian syndrome. Rev Neurol 1965;112:568–79.

[8] Guilleminault C, Tilkian A, Dement WC. The sleep apnea syndromes. Annu Rev Med 1976;27: 465–84.

[9] Young T, Palta M, Dempsey J, et al. The occurrence of sleep-disordered breathing among middle-aged adults. N Engl J Med 1993;328:1230–5.

[10] He J, Kryger MH, Zorick FJ. Mortality and apnea index in obstructive sleep apnea: experience in 385 male patients. Chest 1988;94:9–14.

[11] Shinohara E, Kihara S, Yamashita S, et al. Visceral fat accumulation as an important risk factor for obstructive sleep apnea syndrome in obese subjects. J Intern Med 1997;241:11–8.

[12] Millman RP, Carlisle CC, McGarvey ST, et al. Body fat distribution and sleep apnea severity in women. Chest 1995;107:362–6.

[13] Levenson PD, McGarvey ST, Carlisle CC, et al. Adiposity and cardiovascular risk factors in men with obstructive sleep apnea. Chest 1993;103:1336–42.

[14] Frey WC, Pilcher J. Obstructive sleep-related breathing disorders in patients evaluated for Bariatric surgery. Obes Surg 2003;13:676–83.

[15] O'Keefe T, Patterson EJ. Evidence supporting routine polysomnography before Bariatric surgery. Obes Surg 2004;14:23–6.

[16] Parish JM, Somers VK. Obstructive sleep apnea and cardiovascular disease. Mayo Clin Proc 2004;79:1036–46.

[17] Katz I, Stradling JR, Slutsky AS, et al. Do patients with obstructive sleep apnea have thick neck? Am Rev Respir Dis 1990;141:1228–31.

[18] Strobel RJ, Rosen RC. Obesity and weight loss as a treatment for obstructive sleep apnea: a critical review. Sleep 1996;19:104–15.

[19] Boushra NN. Anesthetic management of patients with sleep apnea syndrome. Can J Anaesth 1996;43:599–616.

[20] Mathew JP, Rosenbaum SH, O'Connor T, et al. Emergency tracheal intubation in the post-anesthesia care unit: physician error or patient disease? Anesth Analg 1990;71:691–7.

[21] Siyam MA, Benhamou D. Difficult endotracheal intubation in patients with sleep apnea syndrome. Anesth Analg 2002;95:1098–102.

[22] Brodsky JB, Lemmens HJ, Brock-Utne JG, et al. Morbid obesity and tracheal intubation. Anesth Analg 2002;94(3):732–6.

[23] Neill AM, Angus SM, Sajkov D, et al. Effects of sleep posture on upper airway stability in patients with obstructive sleep apnea. Am J Respir Crit Care Med 1997;155:199–204.

[24] Gal TJ, Cooperman LH. Hypertension in the immediate postoperative period. Br J Anaesth 1975; 47:70–4.

[25] Abir F, Bell RL. Assessment and management of the obese patient. Crit Care Med 2003; 32(Suppl 4):S87–91.

[26] Terris DJ, Fincher EF, Hanasono MM, et al. Conservation of resources: indications for intensive care monitoring after upper airway surgery on patients with obstructive sleep apnea. Laryngoscope 1998;108(6):784–8.

[27] Knill RL, Moote CA, Skinner MI, et al. Anesthesia with abdominal surgery leads to intense REM sleep during the first postoperative week. Anesthesiology 1990;73:52–61.

[28] Benumof J. Obstructive sleep apnea in the adult obese patient: implications for airway management. J Clin Anesth 2001;13(2):144–56.

[29] Cullen DJ. Obstructive sleep apnea and postoperative analgesia: a potentially dangerous combination. J Clin Anesth 2001;13(2):83–5.

[30] Lamarche Y, Martin R, Reiher J, et al. The sleep apnoea syndrome and epidural morphine. Can Anaesth Soc J 1986;33(2):231–3.

[31] Ostermeier AM, Roizen MF, Hautkappe M, et al. Three sudden postoperative respiratory arrests associated with epidural opioids in patients with sleep apnea. Anesth Analg 1997;85(2):452–60.

[32] Etches RC. Respiratory depression associated with patient-controlled analgesia: a review of eight cases. Can J Anaesth 1994;41(2):125–32.

[33] Wilson JA, Clark JJ. Obesity: impediment to wound healing. Crit Care Nurs Q 2003;26:119–32.

ELSEVIER
SAUNDERS

Anesthesiology Clin N Am
23 (2005) 501–523

ANESTHESIOLOGY
CLINICS OF
NORTH AMERICA

Nonsurgical and Surgical Treatment of Obesity

Patrick J. Neligan, MD[a,*], Noël Williams, MD[b]

[a]Department of Anesthesia, University of Pennsylvania School of Medicine, 3400 Spruce Street,
Philadelphia, PA 19104, USA
[b]Bariatric Surgery Program, Department of Surgery, University of Pennsylvania School of Medicine,
3400 Spruce Street, PA 19104, USA

We are in the midst of an obesity epidemic. Obesity is classified according to body mass index (BMI) (the weight in kilograms divided by the square of the height in meters). A BMI range of 25–29.9 kg/m^2 is classified as overweight; a range of 30–34.9 kg/m^2 is class I obesity; greater than 35 kg/m^2 is class II obesity; and morbidly obese and extreme obesity are associated with a BMI greater than 40 kg/m^2 (class III obesity). To prevent confusion in this discussion, morbid obesity will refer to all patients with a BMI greater than 35 kg/m^2 (classes II and III).

The prevalence of obesity has increased dramatically in the United States over the past 20 years. Between the periods 1988 to 1994 [1] and 1999 to 2000 [2], the prevalence of adult BMI greater than 25 increased from 55.9% to 64.5%; BMI greater than 30 increased from 22.9% to 30.5%; and BMI greater than 40 increased from 2.9% to 4.7% [2]. This latter category consists of 3.1% of men and 6.3% of women [2]. African-American females, individuals who did not complete high school, and those with short stature are particularly at risk for obesity [3]. Morbid obesity is associated with a twofold increase in the relative risk of death (from all causes) compared with the relative risk of death for BMI of 30–32 [4]. Recent estimates are that $70–100 billion or approximately 10% of all health care costs are attributable to treating obesity and obesity-related complications [5].

Simultaneously, the number of bariatric surgical procedures has increased [6,7]. An estimated 103,000 surgeries were performed in 2003, specifically for morbid obesity [6], in addition to operations performed for conditions such as

---

* Corresponding author.
E-mail address: neliganp@uphs.upenn.edu (P.J. Neligan).

back or knee problems, which were related and unrelated (such as pregnancy) to obesity. Consequently, anesthesiologists are seeing an increasing number of morbidly obese patients presenting for surgery, with the potential for increased perioperative morbidity and mortality. This article reviews surgical and non-surgical options in the management of morbidly obese patients.

Nonsurgical management

Morbid obesity is a medical, psychological, and social problem. Initial medical care involves diet, exercise, and behavior modification. Although there are myriad diet programs available, all of them involve a significant reduction in energy intake. Generally, these programs can be divided into low calorie diets (LCD), consisting of 800 to 1500 kcal/day, and very low calorie diets (VLCD), consisting of less than 800 kcal/day. LCD is preferentially recommended over VLCD because of equal efficacy at 1-year, with less risk of nutritional deficiency and greater compliance [8]. LCD has been shown to reduce body weight by an average of 8% and reduce abdominal fat content over a period of 6 months [9]. Interest in high-protein moderate-fat low-carbohydrate diets (such as the Atkins diet) has intensified over the past few years. Low-carbohydrate diets appear to result in a significantly better rate of weight loss (4% absolute difference) over 6 months [10,11] compared with conventional low-calorie low-fat diets; however, this benefit does not persist at 12 months [12].

Diet alone is insufficient to maintain weight loss. Behavioral modification is necessary and should include physical activity. Physical exercise (three to seven sessions per week, lasting 30 to 60 minutes each) can achieve modest weight loss (2%–3% of body weight), independently of dietary therapy [13]. Although cardiorespiratory fitness is improved by exercise, abdominal fat content changes little [9]; therefore, a combination of exercise and diet is necessary to ensure weight loss and weight maintenance.

The objective of behavioral therapy is to assist in overcoming barriers to compliance with dietary therapy or increased physical activity. The current evidence suggests that behavioral therapy, in addition to exercise and diet, produces weight loss of approximately 10% over 4 months to 1 year [9]. However, this intervention must be sustained to prevent the recovery of lost weight. For the majority of overweight and obese patients, the triad of diet, exercise, and behavior therapy is sufficient to reduce cardiovascular risk, but for morbidly obese patients, weight loss in the range of 4% to 6% is inadequate. Consequently, these patients are suitable for second-level pharmacotherapy.

Weight loss drugs may be used as adjuncts to physical exercise and diet therapy in patients with a BMI greater than 30 without concomitant disease or greater than 27 with comorbidity [8]. Weight loss agents should never be prescribed in the absence of concomitant lifestyle modifications. Even the most casual magazine reader or television viewer would be led by infomercials to believe there is a vast array of weight reduction pills on the market. Surprisingly, the majority of these pills are herbal remedies or products containing ephedrine, and only two weight loss drugs are approved by the Food and Drug Administration (FDA), sibutramine HCl monohydrate (Meridia, Abbott Laboratories) and orlistat (Xenical, Roche) (Table 1).

Pharmacotherapy for obesity remains controversial after the "phen-fen" debacle of the 1990s. Fenfluramine and phentermine were approved in the 1970s as individual weight loss drugs. Both drugs are sympathomimetic amines, pharmacologically similar to amphetamine. Fenfluramine increases the level of serotonin in the central nervous system. The exact mechanism of anorexia is unknown. In 1996, an estimated 18 million prescriptions were filled for fenfluramine, dexfenfluramine, or phenteramine in the United States [14]. Weintraub et al [15] first demonstrated that combining low-dose (off label) phentermine with fenfluramine for obese patients, along with exercise, diet, and lifestyle modification, resulted in impressive weight loss over 24 weeks.

In 1997, Connolly et al [14] reported 24 cases of valvular heart disease in women with no previous cardiac history who were taking phen-fen. The histopathologic features were identical to those seen in carcinoid or ergotamine-induced valve disease [14]. The hypothesis was that high circulating levels of serotonin led to valvulopathy. Increasing concerns regarding the association [16] led to an FDA advisory on phen-fen in 1997 (for details, see www.fda.gov/cder/news/phen/phenfen.htm). At that time, there were 33 reports of abnormal valvular morphology and regurgitation involving the mitral, aortic, and tricuspid valves. Half of the patients had associated pulmonary hypertension. After the advisory, fenfluramine and dexfenfluramine were voluntarily withdrawn from the market. A large study [17] of almost 1500 patients who had received dexfenfluramine, the phen-fen combination, or nothing, was completed in 1998. The prevalence rates and relative risk (RR) of aortic regurgitation were 8.9% in the dexfenfluramine group (RR, 2.18; 95% confidence interval [CI], 1.32–3.59), 13.7% in the phen-fen group (RR, 3.34; 95% CI, 2.09–5.35), and 4.1% in the untreated group ($P \leq 0.001$). There was no increase in the risk of mitral regurgitation.

Sibutramine is a serotonin, norepinephrine, and dopamine reuptake inhibitor and works as an appetite suppressant. Sibutramine does not cause valvular heart

Table 1
Food and Drug Administration-approved drugs for weight loss

Drug	Dose	Action	Adverse effects
Sibutramine	5, 10, 15 mg; 10 mg qd orally to start; may be increased to 15 mg or decreased to 5 mg	Norepinephrine, dopamine, and serotonin reuptake inhibitor	Increase in heart rate and blood pressure
Orlistat	120 mg; 120 mg tid orally before meals	Inhibits pancreatic lipase, decrease fat absorption	Decrease in absorption of fat-soluble vitamins; soft stools and anal leakage

Data from Fisher BL, Schauer P. Medical and surgical options in the treatment of severe obesity. Am J Surg 2002;184(Suppl 2):S9–16.

disease. Orlistat binds to ingested fats, preventing intestinal absorption. It acts by forming a covalent bond with the active serine residue site of gastric and pancreatic lipases. The inactivated enzymes are consequently unavailable to hydrolyze dietary fats, so absorption is reduced by 30%. The clinical efficacy of these two agents was evaluated recently by the Cochrane investigators [18]. Eleven orlistat weight loss studies (four of which reported a second-year weight maintenance phase) and five sibutramine studies (three weight loss and two weight maintenance trials) were appraised. Dropout rates averaged 33% during the weight loss phase of orlistat trials and 43% in sibutramine studies. All patients received lifestyle modification therapy as a co-intervention. Orlistat-treated patients lost 2.7 kg (95% CI: 2.3–3.1 kg) or 2.9% more weight (95% CI: 2.3%–3.4%) compared with those receiving placebo. Patients taking sibutramine experienced 4.3 kg (95% CI: 3.6–4.9 kg) or 4.6% greater weight loss (95% CI: 3.8%–5.4%) than those taking placebo. The number of patients who achieved at least 10% weight loss was 12% higher (95% CI: 8%–16%) with orlistat and 15% higher (95% CI: 4%–27%) with sibutramine therapy than with placebo. The major side effects of orlistat are loose, oily stools and fat-soluble vitamin deficiency. Side effects of sibutramine include dry mouth, insomnia, asthenia, constipation, and a small increase in blood pressure and pulse rate [19,20]. The use of sibutramine should be avoided in patients with coronary heart disease. Regaining weight is inevitable within 12 months after the discontinuation of both these agents [19]. Notably, studies of pharmacotherapy for obesity have focused on weight loss rather than improvement in comorbid conditions. It is unclear what medical benefit, if any, exists with these agents.

Bariatric surgery

The surgical treatment of morbid obesity is known as bariatric surgery. As discussed above, morbidly obese patients rarely respond to medical and dietary therapy. Obesity surgery should be considered in adult patients with a documented BMI greater than or equal to 35 and related comorbidity or a BMI of at least 40 (Box 1). Bariatric surgery reduces obesity-related complications and reduces long-term morbidity, mortality, and the use of health care resources [21–24].

The Swedish obese subjects (SOS) studies [25,26] compared different types of obesity surgery with conservative treatment in a matched-pair design. This was a nonrandomized observational trial. Patients with a BMI greater than 34 were studied over 2 years. Significantly greater weight loss was shown after surgical treatment rather than nonsurgical treatment, and this weight loss resulted in significant improvements of comorbidities, such as diabetes (from a baseline prevalence of 19% to 10% after 2 years), hypertension (from 53% to 31%), sleep apnea (from 23% to 8%), dyspnea when climbing stairs (from 87% to 19%), and chest pain when climbing stairs (from 28% to 4%). Patients perceived a significant difference in their quality of life, particularly among women, which

---

Box 1. Indications for bariatric surgery

Patients should meet the following criteria to be considered for bariatric surgery:

- They should have a BMI ≥ 40 kg/m^2 or BMI ≥ 35 kg/m^2 with associated medical comorbidity worsened by obesity
- Failed dietary therapy
- Psychological stability
- Knowledgeable about the operation and its sequelae
- Motivated
- Have medical problems that do not preclude likely survival from surgery

---

was dependent on absolute weight loss. The more weight the patients lost, the greater their sense was of improvement in quality of life. For example, there was a significant difference in quality of life among women with 30- to 40-kg weight loss and those with more than 40-kg weight loss. The authors suggest that bariatric surgery should target the greatest possible weight loss [25,26].

Preoperative preparation

No clear guidelines exist currently for preoperative preparation, and extensive preoperative testing remains controversial. In addition to a careful history and physical examination, a reasonable battery of preoperative tests would investigate for the presence of previously unidentified comorbidities. A complete blood count, electrolyte levels, hemoglobin A_{1c} and urinalysis, chest radiography, electrocardiography, and spirometry should be included. Some authors advocate abdominal ultrasonography to investigate for gallbladder disease [27]. Polysomnography should be performed in patients with a high risk of obstructive sleep apnea. Psychological screening and preparation should be performed. Liver function tests and coagulation studies should be performed to identify occult hepatic disease. Baseline metabolic parameters such as a lipid profile should be performed as should exclusion of diabetes. The preoperative placement of inferior vena caval (IVC) filters to prevent thromboembolism, a common devastating complication, is controversial. Sapala et al [28] have suggested that a BMI greater than 60, truncal obesity, venous stasis disease, and sleep apnea-obesity hypoventilation syndrome, in combination, represent the highest risk factors. Three or more of these risk factors may indicate IVC filter placement, but in the absence of randomized trials and economic analyses, no recommendations can be given.

Overview of surgical procedures

Historically, two distinct surgical approaches to bariatric surgery have evolved: restrictive and malabsorptive procedures (Fig. 1). Restrictive procedures involve the creation of a small gastric pouch, which fills rapidly, leading to early satiety; these procedures include a variety of gastroplasties and adjustable

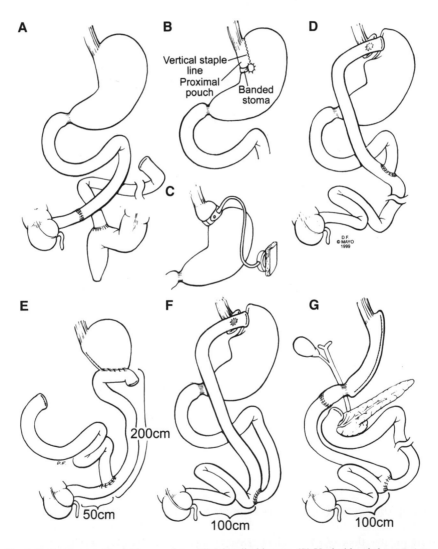

Fig. 1. Past and current bariatric operations. (*A*) Jejunoileal bypass. (*B*) Vertical banded gastroplasty. (*C*) Gastric banding. (*D*) Roux-en-Y gastric bypass. (*E*) Partial biliopancreatic bypass. (*F*) Very long-limb Roux-en-Y gastric bypass. (*G*) Partial biliopancreatic bypass with duodenal switch. (*From* Balsiger, Murr MM, Poggio JL, et al. Surgery for weight control in patients with morbid obesity. Med Clin North Am 2000;84:477–89.)

gastric banding. Malabsorptive procedures involve bypassing a large section of the small bowel, thereby reducing the surface area for absorption. The introduction of high osmolar material into the jejunum leads to a dumping syndrome and avoidance of food. The simpler the procedure is, the greater the likelihood of weight regain, whereas the more complex the procedure is, the more likely complications will ensue.

The first true weight reduction surgery was the jejunoileal bypass, described in 1953, and performed on thousands of patients in the 1960s and 1970s. Although significant weight loss occurred, patients suffered numerous complications associated with malabsorption. Dramatic losses were observed in electrolytes (magnesium and potassium in particular) and water, associated with diarrhea, renal disease, and nephrocalcinosis. In addition, there was significant bacterial overgrowth within the bypassed segment. Liver disease was a particular problem in which one in 12 patients progressed to cirrhosis [29]. The failure of early malabsorptive procedures led to an interest in an alternative approach, a reduction in stomach volume, thus leading to early satiety and reduced food intake (Box 2).

Gastroplasty, which became popular in the 1970s, involves the creation of a 20- to 30-mL pouch in the upper part of the stomach, draining into the main portion. Although a variety of such procedures were performed, only the vertical banded gastroplasty (VBG) procedure described by Mason in 1982 has stood the test of time [30].

The Roux en-Y gastric bypass (RYGB) procedure combines the development of a restrictive pouch and a malabsorptive component, which involves bypassing the duodenum and proximal jejunum. It is the most popular weight loss surgery technique in the United States (Table 2). The RYGB is associated with greater and more sustained weight loss than VBG. Patients also are more prone to

---

Box 2. Bariatric surgical operations mechanism of action

Restrictive

- Vertical banded gastroplasty
- Adjustable gastric banding

Largely restrictive, mildly malabsorptive

- Roux-en-Y gastric bypass

Largely malabsorptive, mildly restrictive

- Biliopancreatic diversion
- Duodenal switch

Table 2
Choice of bariatric procedure for surgeons in the United States and Canada[a]

Operation	Frequency performed (% of total number of procedures)
Roux-en-Y gastric bypass	70
Biliopancreatic diversion	12
Vertical banded gastroplasty	7
Gastric banding	5
Silastic ring gastroplasty	4
Unspecified laparoscopic bariatric surgery	3

[a] American Society of Bariatric Surgery survey, 1999 [31].

postoperative complications (see below). RYGB was performed initially as an open procedure, but surgeons have become interested increasingly in the laparoscopic and hand-assisted approaches.

Malabsorptive surgery re-emerged in the 1990s with the biliopancreatic diversion. Since first being described by Scopinaro et al 30 years ago [32], a modification of this procedure, the duodenal switch, was introduced in the 1990s.

Buchwald and Williams [33] investigated worldwide patterns of bariatric surgery in 2003. During that year, 146,301 bariatric surgery operations were performed by 2839 bariatric surgeons; 103,000 of these operations were performed in United States and Canada by 850 surgeons. The six most popular procedures, according to weighted averages were laparoscopic gastric bypass (25.67%), laparoscopic adjustable gastric banding (24.14%), open gastric bypass (23.07%), laparoscopic long-limb gastric bypass (8.9%), open long-limb gastric bypass (7.45%), and open vertical banded gastroplasty (4.25%). Pooling open and laparoscopic procedures, the relative percentages were gastric bypass, 65.11%; gastric banding, 24.41%; vertical banded gastroplasty, 5.43%; and biliopancreatic diversion and duodenal switch, 4.85%.

Restrictive procedures

The most commonly performed restrictive procedures are VBG and adjustable gastric banding. The former is commonly performed in the United States, whereas the latter is performed commonly in Europe (Box 3).

VBG was first described by Mason at the University of Iowa in 1982. A circular "window" is made through the stomach 6 cm below the gastroesophageal junction. A surgical stapler is then used to create a small vertical pouch by putting a row of staples from the window toward the angle of His. The pouch, which is carefully measured at the time of surgery, will hold approximately 20 mL of solid food. Then, a polypropylene band is placed through the window, around the outlet of the pouch. The band controls the size of the outlet and keeps it from stretching.

Box 3. Complications following vertical banded gastroplasty

Pouch dilatation
Stomal stenosis
Staple line disruption
Stomal ulceration
Incisional hernia
Wound infection
Band erosion

Because of the small size of the gastric pouch, solid food intake is associated with early satiety. Food passing thru the stomach then undergoes normal metabolism. The major advantages of VBG are its relative surgical simplicity, short operative times, and relatively low complication rates. Although the procedure can be performed either as an open procedure or laparoscopically, there is no evidence that the less invasive approach is associated with lower complication rates [34].

The major complications of VBG (see Box 3) include pouch dilatation, stomal stenosis, and the tendency to regain lost weight because the patient adopts high calorie liquid diets. Reoperative rates for VBG are relatively high: the reasons include new-onset gastroesophageal reflux (0.5%–12%), staple-line fistula (0%–3%), food intolerance (0%–2%), outlet stenosis (0%–2%), pouch enlargement (0%–2%), and port-site incisional hernia (0%–0.5%) [34]. The average range of excess weight loss at 3 to 5 years appears to be 30% to 50% [35]. This range deteriorates progressively with time [36]. Interestingly, European patients respond better to gastric restrictive procedures than do US patients [34], but the reason for this difference is unknown.

Two randomized, controlled trials [37,38] have compared laparoscopic with open vertical banded gastroplasty. Both trials documented a longer duration of surgery in the laparoscopic group. The hospital stay was 4 days in both groups in both trials. Respiratory and physical functions recovered more quickly after laparoscopic surgery [38]. Excess weigh loss (EWL) was similar for the two approaches.

Laparoscopic adjustable gastric banding

Laparoscopic adjustable gastric banding (LAGB) is a purely gastric restrictive procedure that involves the use of an adjustable silicone band placed circumferentially around the gastric cardia to create a small gastric pouch (15 mL) with a narrow outlet [39]. This pouch is sutured in place and connected to a subcutaneous port by a small silicone tube. The port is accessed transcutaneously, and saline can be injected or withdrawn from the system, leading to inflation or deflation of the band. Thus the pouch volume can be adjusted.

The LAGB procedure was licensed in the United States in 2001, although the results of an eight-center trial were mixed. Results showed a relatively high incidence of band slippage (23%) and dysphagia, and the surgeon and patient must commit to intensive follow-up for adjustment of the band.

Adjustable gastric banding can be performed as an open or laparoscopic procedure. de Wit et al [40] compared the effectiveness of laparoscopic versus open gastric banding in 50 patients. LAGB was found to be advantageous because of a 1-day reduction in hospital stay and fewer readmissions, although the reduction in BMI was similar. The laparoscopic operation took twice as long (Box 4).

O'Brien et al [41] reported on 4 years of experience with 277 patients who underwent LAGB. The EWL at 1 year was 51%. The weight loss progressed over time to 68.2% at 4 years' follow-up. The operative mortality was 0%, with a 1.8% conversion rate. The main complication was gastric prolapse leading to an increased pouch capacity followed by gastric obstruction (9%).

Angrisani et al [42] reported on 5 years of experience with the LAGB procedure in 1265 patients. The average weight loss at 2 years, reported as a percentage of reduction in the BMI, was 30.8%. The operative mortality was 0.55%, with a 1.7% conversion rate. The major complications cited were pouch dilation (5.2%), band erosion (1.9%), and port or tube problems (4.2%).

Ren et al [43] described outcomes in a 500-patient case series, the majority of which were lost to follow-up. Nevertheless, the percentage of excess weight loss

---

Box 4. Complications following adjustable gastric banding

Operative

    Splenic injury
    Esophageal injury
    Conversion to open procedure
    Wound infection

Postoperative

    Gastric erosion
    Band slippage
    Pouch dilatation
    Reservoir deflation and leakage
    Access port infection
    Failure to lose weight

was 35.6% at 9 months and 41.6% at 12 months. The average body mass index decreased from 47.5 to 38.8 in 9 months and from 47.5 to 37.3 in 12 months. There were no deaths related to the insertion of the device. A total of 15 complications requiring operative management (13%) arose in 12 patients, including eight instances of port displacement or tube breaks (7%), two elective explantations (2%), two cases of gastric prolapse (2%), one gastric pouch dilatation ($\leq$1%), one port abscess ($\leq$1%), and one hemorrhage ($\leq$1%).

LAGB appears to be associated with a mean EWL range of 40% to 60% at 3 to 5 years' follow-up [34,41,44]. The mean hospital stay is less than 2 days, and recovery is rapid. Operative and perioperative mortality rates are very low. Although major complications are uncommon, band slippage (2.2%–10%), port complications (1%–11%), and band erosion (0.3%–1.9%) are the most frequently reported complications that may require reoperation [45,46].

VBG and gastric banding have been compared in three trials, but the studies used different surgical approaches. One trial compared the open version of the procedures [47], one trial compared open VBG with LAGB, [48], and the third trial compared both procedures performed laparoscopically [49]. Taking into account differences in trial design, nonrandomization, and laparoscopic versus open surgery, some conclusions can be drawn. LABG is associated with a shorter hospital stay and fewer early complications. VBG is associated with fewer long-term complications, decreased follow-up requirements, and better weight reduction.

Weber et al [50] compared laparoscopic gastric bypass (L-RYGB) with laparoscopic gastric banding. The study used a matched-pair retrospective approach rather than a randomized design. Mean operating time was significantly shorter for gastric banding, as was the length of hospital stay. There was no difference in the incidence of immediate complications between the groups, but there were significantly less late complications and greater weight loss in the L-RYGB group.

Roux-en-Y gastric bypass

The gastric bypass operation for severe obesity is now the most commonly performed bariatric operation in the United States. Three major variations are the open, laparoscopic, and hand-assisted approaches. The operation is similar: a 15- to 30-mL gastric pouch is created and isolated from the distal stomach by a 21-mm stapled, circular anastomosis (internal diameter 12–14 mm). A 75- to 150-cm ante-colic, ante-gastric Roux limb is created, and a stapled side-to-side jejunojejunostomy is fashioned (Box 5). The purpose of the Roux limb is to divert the pancreatic juice and bile. The longer the Roux limb, the greater the degree of malabsorption.

RYGB should be considered the gold standard of weight loss surgery owing to excellent short-term, intermediate, and long-term weight loss results. Suger-

---

Box 5. Essential components of the Roux-en-Y gastric bypass

A small proximal gastric pouch is created
A gastric pouch is constructed of stomach cardia to prevent
dilation and minimize acid production
The gastric pouch is divided from the distal stomach
A Roux limb of at least 75 cm in length is created
An enteroenterostomy is constructed to avoid stenosis
or obstruction
Closure of all potential spaces for internal hernias

---

man et al [51] followed more than 1025 patients who underwent gastric bypass surgery over a 20-year period. There was a strong correlation between weight loss and the resolution of type 2 diabetes and hypertension. By 1 year after surgery, patients had lost 66% of excess body weight, and hypertension had resolved in 69% and diabetes in 83%. There was a strong relationship between the magnitude of weight loss and the improvement or resolution of comorbidities. This relationship continued with follow-up beyond 5 years. Reddy et al [52] reported a mean excess weight loss of 33% after open RYGB in 103 patients, at a mean follow-up time of 5 months.

Four randomized, controlled trials have compared open RYGB and open vertical banded gastroplasty. Sugerman et al [53] compared results between 20 RYGB and 20 VBG patients at 3 year's follow-up. RYGB showed superior EWL over 1 year (68% versus 43%), but postoperative complications were more common after RYGB. Hall et al [54] found the 3-year EWL to be greater with RYGB than VGB. Howard et al [55] reported greater weight loss with RYGB for up to 5 years, but the patients were not randomized, and follow-up was incomplete. MacLean et al [56] confirmed these results, although the surgical failure rate for VBG was unusually high in this study. Although the traditional open RYGB is effective and results in a relatively low complication rate, surgeons are performing more laparoscopic or modified laparoscopic procedures (Box 6) [57].

Laparoscopic RYGB offers many potential advantages. Incisional hernias occur in 15% to 25% of patients who undergo open RYGB, a complication that is virtually eliminated by the laparoscopic approach. In addition, the incidence of wound infections and other wound-associated complications are reduced. Patients experience less postoperative pain and become ambulatory and leave the hospital earlier. Nevertheless, a steep learning curve is associated with the procedure. In a retrospective analysis of the first 160 patients to undergo laparoscopic Roux-en-Y gastric bypass during a 24-month period, operative time decreased as surgeon experience increased, although the conversion rate, complication rate, and length of stay were not affected by surgeon experience [58]. Weight loss outcomes appear to be similar between the laparoscopic and open

---

Box 6. Complications following Roux en Y gastric bypass

Early

    Anastomotic leakage
    Bleeding
    Acute gastric dilatation
    Roux-en-Y obstruction
    Wound infection and seroma

Late

    Stomal stenosis
    Stomal ulceration

---

approaches at 1-year follow-up (EWL 77 ± 16.7%) [59]. L-RYGB is significantly more difficult than its open counterpart, particularly in superobese patients. As a consequence, a simpler approach, the hand-assisted L-RYGB, has been developed.

L-RYGB was compared with open RYGB in three similarly designed randomized, controlled trials. All studies showed equivalent weight loss for open versus laparoscopic surgery. Nguyen et al [60] reported that hospital lengths of stay were shorter and postoperative complications were fewer in the laparoscopic group. However, a greater incidence of late anastomotic stricture was associated with this approach. Similar results were reported by Westling and Gustavsson [61]. Lujan et al [62] described a shorter duration of surgery and hospital stay for L-RYGB. The incidence of incisional hernia in the open group (10/51) was much higher compared with the laparoscopic group (0/53). Sundbom and Gustavsson [63] compared hand-assisted laparoscopic with open RYGB and found that weight loss was similar in both groups, as were postoperative complications. DeMaria et al [64] confirmed these results in a nonrandomized study. Thus, the technically easier approach of hand-assisted laparoscopy is a good alternative to laparoscopic surgery.

Compared with VBG, a significantly greater risk of complications is associated with RYBG, regardless of the surgical approach [65]. The most significant complication is anastomotic leakage, which is suspected by the development of a systemic inflammatory response, abdominal pain, vomiting, and fluid sequestration. The diagnosis is confirmed by surgery or upper gastrointestinal study.

The most common complications after RYGB involve pulmonary function, principally atelectasis, pneumonia, and pulmonary embolism. Atelectasis can be avoided with preinduction continuous positive airway pressure (CPAP), intraoperative positive end-expiratory pressure, reverse Trendelenburg positioning, and careful postoperative positioning, pulmonary toilet, and CPAP or bilevel positive airway pressure.

Stomal ulceration occurs in one in six patients on the jejunal side of the anastomosis, caused by acid leakage from the gastric remnant [65]. The staple line separating the pouch from the stomach proper may dehisce. A significant long-term risk of bowel obstruction exists from adhesions and internal hernias at the Roux site, the retrocolic window, and between the mesentery and mesocolon.

Particular attention should be paid to the postoperative feeding care of patients undergoing RYGB, who may develop nutrient and micronutrient deficiencies. These include deficiencies of iron, calcium, B_{12}, and folate, which require supplementation. Protein malnutrition is unusual.

Malabsorptive procedures: biliopancreatic diversion

As described originally, the distal two thirds of the stomach is removed, and the 200- 300-mL remnant is connected to the ileum, bypassing the duodenum and jejunum. Therefore, biliopancreatic diversion (BPD) (Fig. 2) is principally a malabsorptive procedure. A common channel remains in which bile and pancreatic digestive juices mix, approximately 50 cm from the ileocecal valve. The flow of food is separated from the flow of digestive juices. Significant weight loss ensues because of malabsorption. However, malabsorption takes place at the expense of a higher incidence of both surgical and metabolic postoperative complications. Patients almost always complain of foul smelling diarrhea. Significant vitamin deficiencies, particularly of vitamins A, D, E, and K, are common. Of particular importance is the development of osteomalacia and secondary hyperparathyroidism caused by vitamin D deficiency.

To overcome the myriad complications associated with BPD, the duodenal switch (DS) was introduced in the 1990s (Fig. 3). In this procedure, the greater curvature of the stomach is excised, leaving the fundus and pyloric valve. The first part of the duodenum is divided and attached to the terminal ileum. Again, a common channel diverts biliary and pancreatic secretions and the jejunum into a common channel 50 cm proximal to the cecum. The advantage of this procedure is the absence of a pouch (the pylorus is spared), which significantly reduces the incidence of dumping syndrome, stomal ulceration, obstruction, and stricture. In addition, the preservation of the early part of the duodenum leads to a reduction in the incidence of vitamin and iron deficiencies. A majority of surgeons who perform BPD now include DS (BPD-DS).

Because of low levels of experience, insurance company remuneration, and concerns regarding long-term complications, BPD is infrequently performed in the United States. Consequently there are few available data comparing BPD with the VBG, LABG, and RYBG procedures.

Rabkin [66] has compared BPD (32 patients), DS (105 patients), and RYGB (138 patients). Follow-up was incomplete, making the validity of the results

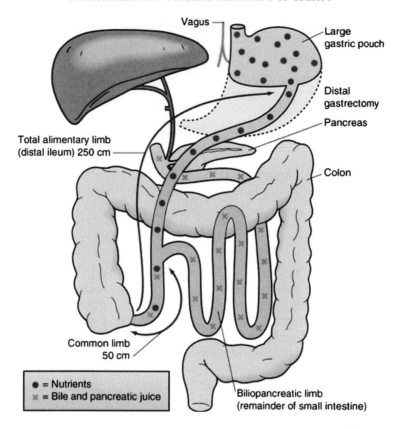

Fig. 2. The duodenal switch procedure. (*From* Marceau P, Hould FS, Lebel S, et al. Malabsorptive obesity surgery. Surg Clin North Am 2001;81:1113–27.)

unclear. A marginally better weight loss was observed with DS than with RYGB (78% versus 74% EWL) at 2 years.

Deveney et al [67] confirmed this equivalence of EWL after BPD and RYGB. It is unclear how the surgeons selected the patients for the specific procedures; selection bias may exist because BMI was greater in patients undergoing BPD-DS. Weight loss and perioperative complications were similar for both groups, although follow-up was incomplete. The average length of stay was longer for BPD-DS patients than for those undergoing RYGB (8.7 versus 5.9 days; $P \leq 0.05$).

Bajardi et al [68] compared BPD with nonadjustable gastric banding (GB). Surgical times and hospital lengths of stay were significantly shorter and complications were fewer after GB. EWL after 2 years was 60% after BPD versus 48% after nonadjustable gastric banding [68]. In a matched-pair analysis, BPD also resulted in greater EWL (64% versus 48%) compared with LAGB [69].

Kalfarentzos et al [70] have studied a cohort of patients undergoing BPD. The mean follow-up time was 29 ± 14 months. Maximum weight loss was

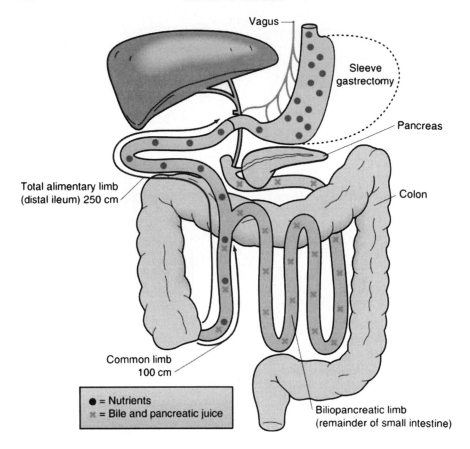

Fig. 3. The biliopancreatic diversion procedure. (*From* Marceau P, Hould FS, Lebel S, et al. Malabsorptive obesity surgery. Surg Clin North Am 2001;81:1113–27.)

achieved at 18 months postoperatively, with an average EWL of 65%, an average initial weight loss of 39%, and an average BMI of 35 kg/m^2. The majority of pre-existing morbidities were permanently resolved by the 6-month follow-up visit. Early mortality was 1%, and early morbidity was 11%. Late morbidity was 27%, half of which was caused by incisional hernia.

Laparoscopic BPD-DS will probably emerge as the surgical approach of choice over time. The first laparoscopic BPD was performed only as recently as 1999 [71,72]. The only comparative study (performed in superobese patients) found similar weight loss and reconvalescence rates after laparoscopic and open BPD but a better improvement rate of comorbidities in the laparoscopic group [73]. This finding, however, should be attributed to different durations of follow-up in the two groups. In summary, the degree of weight loss caused by BPD is greater, compared with alternative approaches, but the weight loss occurs at the expense of increased complication rates.

Future developments

The gastric pacemaker is expected to become a valid therapy for morbid obesity [74,75]. This approach involves the implantation of bipolar electrodes just beneath the seromuscularis of the stomach near the pes anserinus. The electrode is attached to a battery-powered stimulator inserted into a subcutaneous pocket in the upper abdomen. Nerves in the lower stomach are stimulated in pulses at a rate of 12 times per minute, which promotes gastric contraction and induces a feeling of satiety. The mechanism of action is unknown [75]. The pacemaker is individually adjusted to provide maximal anorexia but minimize nausea and vomiting. Efficacy data are currently lacking, although a number of trials are in progress. Faveretti et al [76] reported an EWL of 23.8 $\pm$ 5% at 12 months with this device. It is inserted laparoscopically as an ambulatory procedure, with minimal perioperative complications. The main surgical complication is gastric puncture, which is treated conservatively.

Complications

Postoperative complications may have an atypical presentation in the obese, and early detection and timely management are necessary to prevent deleterious outcomes [77].

After VBG, complications include stoma stenosis, pouch dilatation, band erosion and staple line disruption (see Box 3). Erosion or infection of the band at the pouch outlet should be treated by band removal. Complications after LAGB include gastric erosion, band slippage, pouch dilation, occlusion of the stoma, and port-related complications (see Box 4). Gastric erosion usually causes mild pain and various types of infections and prevents further weight loss. The band should be removed. Band slippage usually presents with heartburn or upper abdominal pain. The band should be deflated. Pouch dilatation is associated usually with weight regain and loss of early satiety. Access ports can twist or become infected, in which case they should be removed. The patient can be converted to RYGB.

The most significant complications of RYBG (Box 6) are anastomotic leakage and bleeding [65]. The presence of fever, tachycardia, and tachypnea after any of these operations should alert the clinician to the possibility of anastomotic leak. A majority of patients can be treated by drainage with or without over-sewing. In some cases, surgery is required to correct the leakage, and this can be performed through an open or a laparoscopic approach. Bleeding usually occurs at the staple line, and it can be treated conservatively. Indeed, a reoperation rarely identifies the source of bleeding. Stomal stenosis caused by anastomotic strictures occurs usually during the first postoperative months [78]. Most cases are amenable to endoscopic dilatation, but some cases require surgical correction for the persistence of stenosis or perforation caused by dilatation.

The complications of BPD are similar to RYGB, with the exception of a significant risk of deficiency in nutrition, vitamins, and trace elements. Patients should be followed by a nutritionist, and supplements should be routinely administered.

Choice of weight loss surgery

Buchwald et al [79] has performed a systematic review of 136 studies, including a total of 22,094 patients. Nineteen percent of the patients were men and 72.6% were women, with a mean age of 39 years (range, 16–64 years). Gender was not reported for 1537 patients (8%). The baseline mean body mass index for 16,944 patients was 46.9 (range, 32.3–68.8). The mean (95% CI) percentage of excess weight loss was 61.2% (58.1%–64.4%) for all patients; 47.5% (40.7%–54.2%) for patients who underwent gastric banding; 61.6% (56.7%–66.5%) for gastric bypass; 68.2% (61.5%–74.8%) for gastroplasty; and 70.1% (66.3%–73.9%) for biliopancreatic diversion or duodenal switch. The operative mortality ($\leq$30 days) in the extracted studies was 0.1% for the purely restrictive procedures, 0.5% for gastric bypass, and 1.1% for biliopancreatic diversion or duodenal switch. Diabetes was completely resolved in 76.8% of patients and resolved or improved in 86.0%. Hyperlipidemia improved in 70% or more of patients. Hypertension was resolved in 61.7% of patients and resolved or improved in 78.5%. Obstructive sleep apnea was resolved in 85.7% of patients and was resolved or improved in 83.6% of patients.

Because obesity surgery has various objectives, such as weight loss, adjustability, reversibility, and safety, there is no optimal bariatric procedure. For all types of surgery, there is evidence from case series on safety, efficacy, and effectiveness in terms of weight loss, but much less data are available on the comparative evaluation of different bariatric procedures. Much of the published data is retrospective, nonrandomized, and flawed by selection bias. Considerable evidence of a direct relationship between the surgical experience and patient outcomes after bariatric surgery is available [80]. Hospital surgical volume is also important. High-volume hospitals (with more than 100 cases annually) show a lower rate of postoperative surgical and medical complications [81].

Intuitively, it might be assumed that the superobese patient and bariatric surgeon would choose the most effective procedure. However, these patients also are at the greatest risk for postoperative complications, in which physiologic reserve is a prime determinant of mortality [82]. Consequently, the surgeon may choose a staged procedure such as VBG or LABG to induce initial weight loss with low complication rates and to correct comorbid conditions, followed 1 or 2 years later by a definitive RYBG or BPD-DS.

Finally, determining the suitability of the patient for surgery is as important as the choice of operation for the individual patient; being merely morbidly obese is insufficient. The patient must have demonstrated an inability to control food intake, expressed a real desire to lose weight, and understand that many major complications are associated with surgery and a significant personal cost is involved. Many bariatric surgeons require preoperative psychological assessment.

Simultaneous surgery

Cholecystectomy has been proposed for all patients (with or without gallstones) at the time of surgery [27]. Many patients have pre-existing gallbladder disease, and obesity surgery promotes postoperative gallstone formation and necessitates subsequent cholecystectomy in approximately 10% of patients [83,84]. Livingston [85] has estimated that 28% of patients undergoing bariatric surgery in the United States undergo cholecystectomy. No clear guidelines are available on this subject; however, patients with pre-existing gallstones, whether symptomatic or asymptomatic, should probably undergo cholecystectomy. The postoperative use of ursodeoxycholic acid has been shown to reduce the risk of subsequent cholecystolithiasis [86].

Follow-up

Patients should be seen three to eight times during the first postoperative year, one to four times during the second year, and once or twice per year thereafter [77]. Specific procedures may require specific follow-up schedules, for example, for an LAGB procedure. Follow-up should involve a surgeon, dietician, psychiatrist, or psychologist.

Summary

Obesity is emerging as one of the greatest health care problem of our time. One in three Americans is now clinically obese. Morbid obesity is associated with a medley of comorbid conditions and poor long-term outcomes. Overweight and obese individuals should be treated with diet, exercise, and behavioral therapy. The failure of this approach is an indication for pharmacologic therapy. Bariatric surgery should be considered in adult patients with a documented BMI greater than or equal to 35 and related comorbidity or a BMI of at least 40 (Table 2). Bariatric surgery reduces obesity-related complications and reduces long-term morbidity, mortality, and health care resources use.

Adjustable gastric banding (AGB), vertical banded gastroplasty (VBG), Roux-en-Y gastric bypass (RYGB), and biliopancreatic diversion (BPD) are all effective procedures in the treatment of morbid obesity. In terms of weight loss, BPD-DS is superior to RYGB, RYGB is superior to AGB, and ABG is superior to VBG. An increased risk of perioperative complications exists in procedures requiring stapling and anastomoses. The reoperation rate is higher for adjustable gastric banding and VBG. There is no ideal bariatric procedure, and because positive and negative effects differ among the procedures, the choice of procedure should be tailored to the patient's BMI, perioperative risk, metabolic situation, comorbidities, and patient and surgeon preference as well as to the surgeon's expertise [77].

References

[1] Kuczmarski RJ, Flegal KM, Campbell SM, et al. Increasing prevalence of overweight among US adults: the National Health and Nutrition Examination Surveys, 1960 to 1991. JAMA 1994; 272:205–11.

[2] Flegal KM, Carroll MD, Ogden CL, et al. Prevalence and trends in obesity among US adults, 1999–2000. JAMA 2002;288:1723–7.

[3] Freedman DS, Khan LK, Serdula MK, et al. Trends and correlates of class 3 obesity in the United States from 1990 through 2000. JAMA 2002;288:1758–61.

[4] Calle EE, Thun MJ, Petrelli JM, et al. Body-mass index and mortality in a prospective cohort of US adults. N Engl J Med 1999;341:1097–105.

[5] Mokdad AH, Bowman BA, Ford ES, et al. The continuing epidemics of obesity and diabetes in the United States. JAMA 2001;286:1195–200.

[6] Steinbrook R. Surgery for severe obesity. N Engl J Med 2004;350:1075–9.

[7] Fernandez Jr AZ, Demaria EJ, Tichansky DS, et al. Multivariate analysis of risk factors for death following gastric bypass for treatment of morbid obesity. Ann Surg 2004;239: 698–702.

[8] Expert Panel on the Identification, Evaluation, and Treatment of Overweight in Adults. Clinical guidelines on the identification, evaluation, and treatment of overweight and obesity in adults: executive summary. Am J Clin Nutr 1998;68:899–917.

[9] Executive summary of the clinical guidelines on the identification, evaluation, and treatment of overweight and obesity in adults. Arch Intern Med 1998;158:1855–67.

[10] Samaha FF, Iqbal N, Seshadri P, et al. Stern et a: A low-carbohydrate as compared with a low-fat diet in severe obesity. N Engl J Med 2003;348:2074–81.

[11] Foster GD, Wyatt HR, Hill JO, et al. A randomized trial of a low-carbohydrate diet for obesity. N Engl J Med 2003;348:2082–90.

[12] Brehm BJ, Seeley RJ, Daniels SR, et al. A randomized trial comparing a very low carbohydrate diet and a calorie-restricted low fat diet on body weight and cardiovascular risk factors in healthy women. J Clin Endocrinol Metab 2003;88:1617–23.

[13] Wood PD, Stefanick ML, Dreon DM, et al. Changes in plasma lipids and lipoproteins in overweight men during weight loss through dieting as compared with exercise. N Engl J Med 1988;319:1173–9.

[14] Connolly HM, Crary JL, McGoon MD, et al. Valvular heart disease associated with fenfluramine-phentermine. N Engl J Med 1997;337:581–8.

[15] Weintraub M, Hasday JD, Mushlin AI, et al. A double-blind clinical trial in weight control: use of fenfluramine and phentermine alone and in combination. Arch Intern Med 1984;144:1143–8.

[16] Bonow RO, Carabello B, de Leon AC, et al. ACC/AHA Guidelines for the management of patients with valvular heart disease: executive summary; a report of the American College of Cardiology/American Heart Association task force on practice guidelines (committee on management of patients with valvular heart disease). J Heart Valve Dis 1998;7:672–707.

[17] Gardin JM, Schumacher D, Constantine G, et al. Valvular abnormalities and cardiovascular status following exposure to dexfenfluramine or phentermine/fenfluramine. JAMA 2000;283: 1703–9.

[18] Padwal R, Li SK, Lau DCW. Long-term pharmacotherapy for obesity and overweight. Cochrane Database Syst Rev 2003;4:CD004094.

[19] Bray GA. Drug treatment of obesity. Rev Endocr Metab Disord 2001;2:403–18.

[20] Fisher BL, Schauer P. Medical and surgical options in the treatment of severe obesity. Am J Surg 2002;184(Suppl 2):S9–16.

[21] Gould JC, Garren MJ, Starling JR. Laparoscopic gastric bypass results in decreased prescription medication costs within 6 months. J Gastrointest Surg 2004;8:983–7.

[22] Christou NV, Sampalis JS, Liberman M, et al. Surgery decreases long-term mortality, morbidity, and health care use in morbidly obese patients. Ann Surg 2004;240:416–23.

[23] Ferchak CV, Meneghini LF. Obesity, bariatric surgery and type 2 diabetes–a systematic review. Diabetes Metab Res Rev 2004;20:438–45.

[24] Anderson JW, Konz EC. Obesity and disease management: effects of weight loss on comorbid conditions. Obes Res 2001;9(Suppl 4):S326–34.

[25] Karlsson J, Sjostrom L, Sullivan M. Swedish obese subjects (SOS)–an intervention study of obesity: two-year follow-up of health-related quality of life (HRQL) and eating behavior after gastric surgery for severe obesity. Int J Obes Relat Metab Disord 1998;22:113–26.

[26] Karason K, Lindroos AK, Stenlof K, et al. Relief of cardiorespiratory symptoms and increased physical activity after surgically induced weight loss: results from the Swedish Obese Subjects study. Arch Intern Med 2000;160:1797–802.

[27] Fobi M, Lee H, Igwe D, et al. Prophylactic cholecystectomy with gastric bypass operation: incidence of gallbladder disease. Obes Surg 2002;12:350–3.

[28] Sapala JA, Wood MH, Schuhknecht MP, et al. Fatal pulmonary embolism after bariatric operations for morbid obesity: a 24-year retrospective analysis. Obes Surg 2003;13:819–25.

[29] Livingston EH. Obesity and its surgical management. Am J Surg 2002;184:103–13.

[30] Mason EE. Vertical banded gastroplasty. Arch Surg 1982;117:701–6.

[31] Schauer PR, Ikramuddin S. Laparoscopic surgery for morbid obesity. Surg Clin North Am 2001;81:1145–79.

[32] Scopinaro N, Gianetta E, Civalleri D. Biliopancreatic bypass for obesity II. Initial experiences in man. Br J Surg 1979;66:618–20.

[33] Buchwald H, Williams SE. Bariatric surgery worldwide 2003. Obes Surg 2004;14:1157–64.

[34] Schauer PR, Ikramuddin S. Laparoscopic surgery for morbid obesity. Surg Clin North Am 2001;81:1145–79.

[35] Sugerman HJ, Starkey JV, Birkenhauer R. A randomized prospective trial of gastric bypass versus vertical banded gastroplasty for morbid obesity and their effects on sweets versus non-sweets eaters. Ann Surg 1987;205:613–24.

[36] MacLean LD, Rhode BM, Forse RA. Late results of vertical banded gastroplasty for morbid and super obesity. Surgery 1990;107:20–7.

[37] Azagra JS, Goergen M, Ansay J, et al. Laparoscopic gastric reduction surgery: preliminary results of a randomized, prospective trial of laparoscopic vs open vertical banded gastroplasty. Surg Endosc 1999;13:555–8.

[38] Davila-Cervantes A, Borunda D, Dominguez-Cherit G, et al. Open versus laparoscopic vertical banded gastroplasty: a randomized controlled double blind trial. Obes Surg 2002;12:812–8.

[39] Belachew M, Legrand M, Vincent V, et al. Laparoscopic adjustable gastric banding. World J Surg 1998;22:955–63.

[40] de Wit LT, Mathus-Vliegen L, Hey C, et al. Open versus laparoscopic adjustable silicone gastric banding: a prospective randomized trial for treatment of morbid obesity. Ann Surg 1999; 230:800–5.

[41] O'Brien PE, Brown WA, Smith A, et al. Prospective study of a laparoscopically placed, adjustable gastric band in the treatment of morbid obesity. Br J Surg 1999;86:113–8.

[42] Angrisani L, Alkilani M, Basso N, et al. Laparoscopic Italian experience with the Lap-Band. Obes Surg 2001;11:307–10.

[43] Ren CJ, Horgan S, Ponce J. US experience with the LAP-BAND system. Am J Surg 2002; 184(Suppl 2):S46–50.

[44] Belachew M, Belva PH, Desaive C. Long-term results of laparoscopic adjustable gastric banding for the treatment of morbid obesity. Obes Surg 2002;12:564–8.

[45] Dargent J. Laparoscopic adjustable gastric banding: lessons from the first 500 patients in a single institution. Obes Surg 1999;9:446–52.

[46] Weiner R, Wagner D, Bockhorn H. Laparoscopic gastric banding for morbid obesity. J Laparo-endosc Adv Surg Tech A 1999;9:23–30.

[47] Nilsell K, Thorne A, Sjostedt S, et al. Prospective randomised comparison of adjustable gastric banding and vertical banded gastroplasty for morbid obesity. Eur J Surg 2001;167:504–9.

[48] Ashy AR, Merdad AA. A prospective study comparing vertical banded gastroplasty versus laparoscopic adjustable gastric banding in the treatment of morbid and super-obesity. Int Surg 1998;83:108–10.

[49] Morino M, Toppino M, Bonnet G, et al. Laparoscopic adjustable silicone gastric banding versus vertical banded gastroplasty in morbidly obese patients: a prospective randomized controlled clinical trial. Ann Surg 2003;238:835–41.

[50] Weber M, Muller MK, Bucher T, et al. Laparoscopic gastric bypass is superior to laparoscopic gastric banding for treatment of morbid obesity. Ann Surg 2004;240:975–82.

[51] Sugerman HJ, Wolfe LG, Sica DA, et al. Diabetes and hypertension in severe obesity and effects of gastric bypass-induced weight loss. Ann Surg 2003;237:751–6.

[52] Reddy RM, Riker A, Marra D, et al. Open Roux-en-Y gastric bypass for the morbidly obese in the era of laparoscopy. Am J Surg 2002;184:611–5.

[53] Sugerman HJ, Starkey JV, Birkenhauer R. A randomized prospective trial of gastric bypass versus vertical banded gastroplasty for morbid obesity and their effects on sweets versus non-sweets eaters. Ann Surg 1987;205:613–24.

[54] Hall JC, Watts JM, O'Brien PE, et al. Gastric surgery for morbid obesity: the Adelaide Study. Ann Surg 1990;211:419–27.

[55] Howard L, Malone M, Michalek A, et al. Gastric bypass and vertical banded gastroplasty: a prospective randomized comparison and 5-year follow-up. Obes Surg 1995;5:55–60.

[56] MacLean LD, Rhode BM, Sampalis J, et al. Results of the surgical treatment of obesity. Am J Surg 1993;165:155–60.

[57] Wittgrove AC, Clark GW. Laparoscopic gastric bypass, Roux-en-Y: experience of 27 cases, with 3–18 months follow-up. Obes Surg 1996;6:54–7.

[58] Kligman MD, Thomas C, Saxe J. Effect of the learning curve on the early outcomes of laparoscopic Roux-en-Y gastric bypass. Am Surg 2003;69:304–9.

[59] Schauer PR, Ikramuddin S, Gourash W, et al. Outcomes after laparoscopic Roux-en-Y gastric bypass for morbid obesity. Ann Surg 2000;232:515–29.

[60] Nguyen NT, Goldman C, Rosenquist CJ, et al. Laparoscopic versus open gastric bypass: a randomized study of outcomes, quality of life, and costs. Ann Surg 2001;234:279–89.

[61] Westling A, Gustavsson S. Laparoscopic vs open Roux-en-Y gastric bypass: a prospective, randomized trial. Obes Surg 2001;11:284–92.

[62] Lujan JA, Frutos MD, Hernandez Q, et al. Laparoscopic versus open gastric bypass in the treatment of morbid obesity: a randomized prospective study. Ann Surg 2004;239:433–7.

[63] Sundbom M, Gustavsson S. Randomized clinical trial of hand-assisted laparoscopic versus open Roux-en-Y gastric bypass for the treatment of morbid obesity. Br J Surg 2004;91:418–23.

[64] DeMaria EJ, Schweitzer MA, Kellum JM, et al. Hand-assisted laparoscopic gastric bypass does not improve outcome and increases costs when compared to open gastric bypass for the surgical treatment of obesity. Surg Endosc 2002;16:1452–5.

[65] Byrne TK. Complications of surgery for obesity. Surg Clin North Am 2001;81:1181–93.

[66] Rabkin RA. Distal gastric bypass/duodenal switch procedure, Roux-en-Y gastric bypass and biliopancreatic diversion in a community practice. Obes Surg 1998;8:53–9.

[67] Deveney CW, MacCabee D, Marlink K, et al. Roux-en-Y divided gastric bypass results in the same weight loss as duodenal switch for morbid obesity. Am J Surg 2004;187:655–9.

[68] Bajardi G, Ricevuto G, Mastrandrea G, et al. Surgical treatment of morbid obesity with biliopancreatic diversion and gastric banding: report on an 8-year experience involving 235 cases. Ann Chir 2000;125:155–62 [in Italian].

[69] Doldi SB, Micheletto G, Perrini MN, et al. Intragastric balloon: another option for treatment of obesity and morbid obesity. Hepatogastroenterology 2004;51:294–7.

[70] Kalfarentzos F, Papadoulas S, Skroubis G, et al. Prospective evaluation of biliopancreatic diversion with Roux-en-Y gastric bypass in the super obese. J Gastrointest Surg 2004;8:479–88.

[71] Ren CJ, Patterson E, Gagner M. Early results of laparoscopic biliopancreatic diversion with duodenal switch: a case series of 40 consecutive patients. Obes Surg 2000;10:514–23.

[72] Davila-Cervantes A, Borunda D, Dominguez-Cherit G, et al. Open versus laparoscopic vertical banded gastroplasty: a randomized controlled double blind trial. Obes Surg 2002;12:812–8.

[73] Kim WW, Gagner M, Kini S, et al. Laparoscopic vs. open biliopancreatic diversion with duodenal switch: a comparative study. J Gastrointest Surg 2003;7:552–7.

[74] De Luca M, Segato G, Busetto L, et al. Progress in implantable gastric stimulation: summary of results of the European multi-center study. Obes Surg 2004;14(Suppl 1):S33–9.

[75] Cigaina V. Gastric pacing as therapy for morbid obesity: preliminary results. Obes Surg 2002; 12(Suppl 1):S12–6.

[76] Favretti F, De Luca M, Segato G, et al. Treatment of morbid obesity with the Transcend Implantable Gastric Stimulator (IGS): a prospective survey. Obes Surg 2004;14:666–70.

[77] Sauerland S, Angrisani L, Belachew M, et al. Obesity surgery: evidence-based guidelines of the European Association for Endoscopic Surgery (EAES). Surg Endosc 2004 Dec 2.

[78] Sanyal AJ, Sugerman HJ, Kellum JM, et al. Stomal complications of gastric bypass: incidence and outcome of therapy. Am J Gastroenterol 1992;87:1165–9.

[79] Buchwald H, Avidor Y, Braunwald E, et al. Bariatric surgery: a systematic review and meta-analysis. JAMA 2004;292:1724–37.

[80] Flum DR, Dellinger EP. Impact of gastric bypass operation on survival: a population-based analysis. J Am Coll Surg 2004;199:543–51.

[81] Nguyen NT, Paya M, Stevens CM, et al. The relationship between hospital volume and outcome in bariatric surgery at academic medical centers. Ann Surg 2004;240:586–93.

[82] Helling TS, Willoughby TL, Maxfield DM, et al. Determinants of the need for intensive care and prolonged mechanical ventilation in patients undergoing bariatric surgery. Obes Surg 2004;14: 1036–41.

[83] Shiffman ML, Sugerman HJ, Kellum JM, et al. Gallstone formation after rapid weight loss: a prospective study in patients undergoing gastric bypass surgery for treatment of morbid obesity. Am J Gastroenterol 1991;86:1000–5.

[84] Jones Jr KB. Simultaneous cholecystectomy: to be or not to be. Obes Surg 1995;5:52–4.

[85] Livingston EH. Procedure incidence and in-hospital complication rates of bariatric surgery in the United States. Am J Surg 2004;188:105–10.

[86] Wudel Jr LJ, Wright JK, Debelak JP, et al. Prevention of gallstone formation in morbidly obese patients undergoing rapid weight loss: results of a randomized controlled pilot study. J Surg Res 2002;102:50–6.

ELSEVIER
SAUNDERS

Anesthesiology Clin N Am
23 (2005) 525–534

ANESTHESIOLOGY
CLINICS OF
NORTH AMERICA

Nonsurgical and Surgical Treatments for Sleep Apnea

Marion Everett Couch, MD, PhD*, Brent Senior, MD

*Department of Otolaryngology–Head and Neck Surgery,
University of North Carolina School of Medicine, G0412 Neurosciences Hospital,
CB 7070, Chapel Hill, NC 27599-7070, USA*

Untreated obstructive sleep apnea (OSA) introduces increased risks to anesthesia and surgery [1]. From the initial management of the airway to the increased incidence of stroke and myocardial infarction, the management of patients with OSA has important implications for the anesthesiologist. OSA should be suspected in patients with large tonsils, a large tongue, poor nasal airway, an edematous uvula, a small mandible (often disguised by a beard in males), a collar size greater than 17 inches, and obesity [1]. Treatment is based on relieving the various levels of obstruction. Modern surgical management of OSA is designed to create site-specific alterations of the upper airway to eliminate airway obstruction. This article reviews the various treatments currently available for OSA and discusses some newer and more controversial therapies.

Nonsurgical treatments

Continuous positive airway pressure

Continuous positive airway pressure (CPAP) remains the recommended initial treatment for OSA. The American Academy of Sleep Medicine guidelines [2] recommend CPAP treatment for patients with an apnea index (AI) (mean number of apneic episodes per hour while sleeping) greater than 20 and for symptomatic

---

* Corresponding author.
E-mail address: marion_couch@med.unc.edu (M.E. Couch).

patients with an apnea-hypopnea index (AHI) (mean number of apneic and hypopneic episodes per hour of sleep) of greater than 10.

The proper use of nasal CPAP will effectively eliminate excessive daytime sleepiness and will reduce hypertension [3]. Improved neurocognitive function is found after adequate CPAP therapy [2]. Long-term use (greater than 18 months) is associated with significant improvement in many health-related quality of life parameters such as improvement in vitality, general health perception, and social and physical functioning [4]. It is believed to function as a mechanical stent of the airway. In addition, the increased augmentation of lung volume by CPAP may elicit a reflex that increases the tone of the upper airway muscles involved with dilation, but this theory is controversial [2].

The effects of adequate CPAP therapy on the cardiovascular system have been substantiated by many studies [2]. Left ventricular failure is improved by CPAP [5]. CPAP treatment for patients with congestive heart failure reduces morbidity and is associated with improved New York Heart Association functional class [6]. A reduction in the sympathetic tone may be the mechanism by which CPAP improves cardiovascular outcomes [2].

Bilevel positive airway pressure (bilevel PAP) allows for improved patient comfort while providing ventilatory assistance for patients who require high CPAP. Independent adjustment of the inspiratory and expiratory airway pressures allows for a possible decrease in the expiratory pressure while providing adequate inspiratory airway pressure. In patients who require high CPAP settings, such as those with chronic obstructive pulmonary disease, exhaling against high positive pressure is difficult. Bilevel PAP is one way of improving tolerance [2].

Although nasal CPAP is highly effective and found to be acceptable in 72% to 91% of those for whom it is prescribed, many patients do not tolerate the equipment. Some equipment is bulky, noisy, difficult to bring on trips, and requires electricity. Not all patients will be able to sleep on their backs and may knock the mask off. These devices create social stigmas for single people and can elicit intolerance by the patient's partner. The mask must also fit well, and despite a good fit, some patients can simply not tolerate masks because of claustrophobia, nasal congestion, rhinorrhea, chest discomfort, and inconvenience. Therefore, adherence to CPAP is often a separate issue from acceptance [2], and indeed, a noncompliance rate of 10% to 50% is widely recognized. If noncompliance ensues, other approaches should be investigated, but nasal CPAP remains as the cornerstone of therapy, with only select patients benefiting from other forms of therapy [7].

Adjustable oral appliances

Mandibular repositioning devices (MRDs) are believed to be effective because they advance the mandible 5 to 6 mm forward, which moves the tongue base anteriorly in a manner analogous to the jaw thrust technique. The primary role of MRDs is to provide a treatment for patients with snoring or mild to moderate OSA. Also, if a patient is unable to tolerate CPAP, the American Sleep Disorders

Association currently recommends they try dental appliances. It may be an acceptable alternative treatment for certain patients with severe OSA [8]. In a recent review [9], oral appliances were less effective than CPAP in reducing the apnea-hypopnea index, but there was evidence to suggest that oral appliances improved subjective sleepiness and sleep disordered breathing.

Compliance is high (50%–75%) but can become an issue because xerostomia, dental pain, temporomandibular joint pain, excessive salivation, and changes in occlusion may result. A majority of patients will experience at least one of these side effects [10].

Weight loss and behavioral therapies

Obesity is common among patients with severe OSA. A body mass index (BMI) of greater than 25 kg/m^2 was found to be a marker for severe OSA [1]. OSA often may be cured by surgical weight loss or with sufficient life-style modifications, but without long-term weight management, the OSA will return [11].

The importance of positioning during sleep was demonstrated by the use of a triangular pillow that had space for the patient's arm under the head to encourage sleeping on the side. The use of the pillow was effective in significantly reducing the respiratory disturbance index (RDI) in patients with mild to moderate sleep apnea [12]. More mundane recommendations include taping a tennis ball to the back of the pajamas to encourage sleeping on the side.

Surgical treatments

Before surgery can be considered, a complete evaluation of each patient is mandatory. This evaluation includes a recent polysomnogram to assess the severity of the OSA. A thorough head and neck examination usually includes a flexible nasopharyngolaryngeal fiber-optic examination along with a careful assessment of possible areas of disproportionate anatomy. It is important to note the presence of an elongated soft palate, thickened uvula (Fig. 1), a large base of the tongue, a deviated nasal septum, enlarged tonsils, hypertrophic nasal turbinates, and a hypoplastic or retrognathic mandible. Imaging studies such as cephalometrics or a CT scans may complement the physical examination findings, as well [13]. Recommendations for possible surgery should be based on relieving site-specific problems in the upper airway.

Uvulopharyngopalatoplasty

Uvulopharyngopalatoplasty (UPPP), removal of a rim of the soft palate and the uvula, was first described in 1964 as a treatment for snoring. Subsequently, Fujita described applying UPPP for the treatment of OSA with a successful outcome [14]. Often, while trimming excess palatal length and an enlarged, thick-

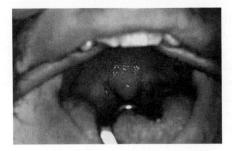

Fig. 1. Typical appearance of the oropharynx in patients with obstructive sleep apnea. Note the elongated palate and uvula with mucosal folding and furrowing over the uvula.

ened uvula, a tonsillectomy is combined with this procedure. The resulting anatomic effect is to enlarge the oropharyngeal airway (Fig. 2). The overall success rate in curing patients of OSA is approximately 40% to 50% (defined as a drop in the RDI ≥50% or an absolute RDI ≤20), but the success rate drops if retrolingual narrowing from either an enlarged tongue or crowding in the region of the hypopharynx is present [15]. Interestingly, the success rates do not increase in the presence of mild OSA [16]. It is the most common surgical procedure performed for OSA and is relatively safe, with an incidence of serious nonfatal complications and mortality of 1.5% and 0.2%, respectively [17]. In a study [18] of perioperative complications and risk factors in the surgical treatment of obstructive sleep apnea syndrome, airway problems comprised 77% of the complications and resulted in one death.

Tonsillectomy

A common area of airway blockage is the palatine tonsils. Removal of the tonsils for tonsillar hypertrophy often offers substantial improvement in airflow

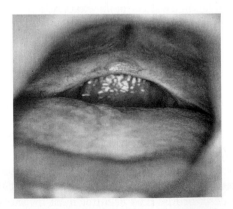

Fig. 2. Typical appearance of the oropharynx after UPPP. The elongated palate has been shortened and the uvula removed. The tonsils also have been removed and the tonsillar pillars narrowed.

in the posterior pharyngeal area. A study [19] of surgical response, defined as a decrease in the postoperative AHI to less than 50%, showed a rate of 80% in severe apneic adults and 100% for patients with mild apnea. Tonsillectomy is a major treatment modality with children, especially when combined with adenoidectomy. It also represents an accepted surgical procedure for adults [20].

Less painful and less invasive procedures to reduce the tonsillar tissue, including the use of temperature-controlled radiofrequency tissue ablation, are being investigated. This technique may be performed with local anesthesia in the office setting or in the operating room. A probe is placed into the tonsils, and volumetric tissue reduction occurs as a result of scarring from the administration of radio-wave energy to the tissue. An initial randomized study [21] found reduced pain when this technique was compared with standard electrocautery. Electrocautery may be combined with radiofrequency tissue ablation of other levels of obstruction, such as the soft palate or tongue base, to improve daytime somnolence and polysomnographic respiratory parameters [22]. Initial reports [23–25] suggest that temperature-controlled radiofrequency tissue ablation is not only safe but it is effective in reducing tonsillar tissue for at least 1 year.

Nasal surgery

Nasal surgery may be recommended to improve compliance with nasal CPAP, especially after maximal medial therapy for nasal obstruction caused by a deviated nasal septum, allergic rhinitis, nasal polyposis, or chronic rhinosinusitis. Procedures such as septoplasty and turbinate reduction are often considered as adjuncts to other surgical procedures because increased nasal resistance or obstruction may increase the negative pressure of the airway during inspiration, which may result in the collapse of the velopharyngeal area and the hypopharyngeal regions [13]. Unfortunately, outcome data on the clinical usefulness is controversial; for example, one study [26] found that straightening the deviated nasal septum with a septoplasty procedure actually worsened OSA.

Tracheostomy

The first surgical procedure proposed for the treatment of severe OSA remains the only surgical procedure that will consistently cure patients with severe OSA. The indications for performing a tracheostomy are the presence of life-threatening, severe OSA and the inability to tolerate CPAP. Alternatively, if CPAP is incapable of effectively overcoming severe deoxygenation or hypercapnia and related symptoms, a tracheostomy may represent the only way to eliminate the OSA. The placement of a tracheostomy tube or the creation of a more permanent skin-lined tracheotomy often results in profound improvement of the patient's OSA [27]. However, in patients with OSA complicated by cardiopulmonary decomposition, a tracheotomy improved but did not completely eliminate the OSA [28]. Therefore, certain patient populations, such as those with a Pickwickian body habitus, may still require nighttime ventilatory support even with the tracheostomy in place. Thus, postoperative sleep studies may be valuable for selected patients with OSA and other serious comorbidities [28].

Jaw advancement techniques

Orthognathic surgery is recommended for patients with pharyngeal or hypopharyngeal narrowing that cannot be adequately addressed by UPPP, tonsillectomy, or minimally invasive procedures such as genioglossus advancement and hyoid suspension (see below). This more radical surgical approach is effective for enlarging the posterior airway. Surgeons create Le Fort I and bilateral mandibular osteotomies to move the tongue and entire midface forward, typically approximately 10 mm. Although success rates as high as 97% have been reported with this procedure [29], this skeletal advancement technique has the potential to alter the patient's facial appearance, and this must be weighed against the potential improvements in sleep parameters. These procedures may be performed in conjunction with other surgeries, such as UPPP, and may be part of a series of planned, staged procedures [15]. More outcomes studies are needed to determine which patients will truly benefit from these procedures.

Minimally invasive techniques

Genioglossus advancement

To address retropalatal and retrolingual airway obstruction, a new procedure uses a guided trephine system to advance the genioglossus muscle forward (Fig. 3). It is often performed in conjunction with UPPP. A recent study [30] demonstrated a 67% surgical success rate, defined by a reduction of greater than 50% in the respiratory disturbance rate and apnea indexes. The posterior airway was significantly increased, as well. Long-term success rates are still being determined.

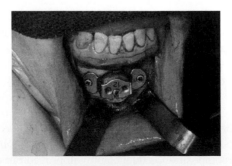

Fig. 3. Intraoperative view showing the genioglossus advancement procedure using a trephine technique. The advanced fragment is secured with a plate.

Tongue-base suspension

For tongue-based obstructive sleep apnea, a minimally invasive tongue-base suspension has been designed to counteract the tongue-base collapse. A titanium screw is inserted into the posterior aspect of the mandible at the floor of the mouth. A loop of permanent suture extending through the tongue base is attached to the mandibular bone screw. This suture loop acts to suspend the tongue base, thereby decreasing the posterior obstruction of the tongue base during sleep. Advocates tout the ability of this procedure to be performed in conjunction with other procedures such as UPPP for OSA. In addition, the tongue-base suspension procedure is potentially reversible. However, the surgical cure rate is controversial. A recent study [31] found that only 20% of patients were cured. Long-term outcomes studies will be needed to determine the success rate.

Multilevel radiofrequency tissue ablation

For patients who have multilevel obstruction, especially at the level of the tongue base and soft palate, temperature-controlled radiofrequency tissue ablation may be an acceptable treatment. In a recent study [32], patients with mild to severe OSA, without tonsil hypertrophy, underwent multiple treatment sessions. All of the procedures were performed in the office with local anesthesia. Pretreatment and post-treatment polysomnograms were compared. This treatment was found to significantly improve the AHI and AI. On average, the patients enjoyed increased quality of life and normalization of their daytime somnolence. Another study [33] documented the absence of postprocedural complications or changes in functional parameters of the sites treated. Although temperature-controlled radiofrequency tissue ablation is promising, large scale, randomized prospective studies are needed to confirm the effectiveness of this treatment.

Future surgical research: physiotherapy of lingual and supra-hyoid muscles

In some pilot studies [34], apneic patients have undergone muscle strengthening with transcutaneous neuromuscular stimulation to counteract muscle dysfunction that may be contributing to the collapse of the upper airway. Preliminary work is intriguing, but larger studies with longer follow-up are needed.

Perioperative issues for obstructive sleep apnea surgery

Presently, it remains controversial whether an overnight stay in a hospital or in a monitored setting within the hospital is necessary after surgery for OSA. A recent study [35] of patients undergoing UPPP found that respiratory events such as airway obstruction, laryngospasm, desaturation, and postobstructive pulmonary edema occurred in 2% to 11% of cases. Postoperative hemorrhage occurred in 2% to 14% of cases and usually occurred immediately or several days after surgery. Hypertension was most common and was seen in 2% to 70% of patients, usually in the immediate postoperative setting. Because a majority of complications occurred within 2 hours of surgery, it was recommended that careful postoperative monitoring would be sufficient to ensure that patients are experiencing no complications and are able to maintain preoperative saturations. However, the degree of OSA along with the extent of surgery must be carefully considered for each patient. For instance, combining UPPP with extensive nasal surgery requiring nasal packing may predispose a patient with OSA to an increased risk of airway obstruction and postoperative hemorrhage. Indeed, an association has been found between the development of complications and operations consisting of multiple simultaneous procedures, such as UPPP combined with septoplasty, tonsillectomy, turbinate reduction, and tracheostomy [36]. Additionally, the amount of narcotics that are administered intraoperatively has been found to be a risk factor for predicting postoperative complications [18].

Summary

The cornerstone of treatment for OSA remains nasal CPAP. For patients who prefer to avoid using a device each night or for those who are unable to tolerate it, there are many surgical and nonsurgical options. Decisions regarding the best treatment should be aimed at relieving the unique levels of obstruction in each patient. More randomized controlled outcome trials will be needed to assess the success of each therapy in certain subpopulations in comparison with CPAP. As these data become available, the roles of each therapy will become clearer in treating this major health problem.

References

[1] Hillman DR, Loadsman JA, Platt PR, et al. Obstructive sleep apnoea and anaesthesia. Sleep Med Rev 2004;8(6):459–71.

[2] Gordon P, Sanders M. Sleep 7: positive airway pressure therapy for obstructive sleep apnoea/hypopnoea syndrome. Thorax 2005;60:68–75.

[3] Jenkinson C, Davies R, Mullins R, et al. Long-term benefits in self-reported health status of nasal continuous positive airway pressure therapy for obstructive sleep apnoea. J Assoc Physicians India 2001;94(2):95–9.

[4] Pichel F, Zamarron C, Magan F, et al. Health-related quality of life in patients with obstructive sleep apnea: effects of long-term positive airway pressure treatment. Respir Med 2004;89(10): 968–76.

[5] Garpestad E, Katayama H, Parker J, et al. Stroke volume and cardiac output decrease at termination of obstructive apneas. J Appl Physiol 1992;73:1743–8.

[6] Sin D, Logan A, Fitzgerald F, et al. Effects of continuous positive airway pressure on cardiovascular outcomes in heart failure patients with and without Cheyne-Stokes respiration. Circulation 2000;119:1092–101.

[7] Chhajed P, Chhajed T, Tamm M, et al. Obstructive sleep apnea: therapies other than CPAP. J Assoc Physicians India 2004;52:143–51.

[8] Walker-Engstrom M, Tegelberg A, Wilhelmsson B, et al. 4-year follow-up of treatment with dental appliance of uvulopalatopharyngoplasty in patients with obstructive sleep apnea: a randomized study. Chest 2002;121(3):739–46.

[9] Lim J, Lasserson T, Fleetham J, et al. Oral appliances for obstructive sleep apnea. Cochrane Database Syst Rev 2004;18(4):CD004435.

[10] Counter P, Wilson J. The treatment of snoring. ENT News 2004;13(4):45–7.

[11] Gami A, Caples S, Somers V. Obesity and obstructive sleep apnea. Endocrinol Metab Clin North Am 2003;32(4):869–94.

[12] Zuberi N, Rekab K, Nguyen H. Sleep apnea avoidance pillow effects on obstructive sleep apnea syndrome and snoring. Sleep Breath 2004;8(4):201–7.

[13] Aragon S. Surgical management for snoring and sleep apnea. Dent Clin North Am 2001; 45(4):867–79.

[14] Fujita S, Conway W, Zorick F, et al. Surgical correction of anatomic abnormalities in obstructive sleep apnea syndrome: uvulopalatopharyngoplasty. Otolaryngol Head Neck Surg 1981;89(6): 923–34.

[15] Bettega G, Pepin J, Veale D, et al. Obstructive sleep apnea syndrome: fifty-one consecutive patients treated by maxillofacial surgery. Am J Respir Crit Care Med 2000;162(2):641–9.

[16] Senior B, Rosenthal L, Lumley A, et al. Effectiveness of uvulopalatopharyngoplasty in un-selected patients for mild obstructive sleep apnea. Otolaryngol Head Neck Surg 2000;123(3): 179–82.

[17] Kezirian E, Weaver E, Yueh B, et al. Incidence of serious complications after uvulopalatophya-ryngoplasty. Laryngoscope 2004;114(3):450–3.

[18] Esclamado R, Glenn M, McCulloch T, et al. Perioperative complications and risk factors in the surgical treatment of obstructive sleep apnea syndrome. Laryngoscope 1989;99(11): 1125–9.

[19] Verse T, Kroker B, Pirsig W, et al. Tonsillectomy as a treatment of obstructive sleep apnea in adults with tonsillar hypertrophy. Laryngoscope 2000;110(9):1556–9.

[20] Guilleminuault C, Abad V. Obstructive sleep apnea. Curr Treat Options Neurol 2004;6(4): 309–17.

[21] Hall D, Littlefield P, Birkmire-Peters D, et al. Radiofrequency ablation versus electrocautery in tonsillectomy. Otolaryngol Head Neck Surg 2004;130(3):300–5.

[22] Fischer Y, Khan M, Mann W. Multilevel temperature-controlled radiofrequency therapy of soft palate, base of tongue, and tonsils in adults with obstructive sleep apnea. Laryngoscope 2003; 113(10):1786–91.

[23] Friedman M, LoSavio P, Ibrahim H, et al. Radiofrequency tonsil reduction: safety, morbidity, and efficacy. Laryngoscope 2003;113(5):882–7.

[24] Nelson L. Temperature-controlled radiofrequency tonsil reduction: extended follow-up. Oto-laryngol Head Neck Surg 2001;125(5):456–61.

[25] Nelson L. Radiofrequency treatment for obstructive tonsillar hypertrophy. Arch Otolaryngol Head Neck Surg 2000;126(6):736–40.

[26] Friedman M, Ibrahim H, Joseph N. Staging of obstructive sleep apnea/hypopnea syndrome: a guide to appropriate treatment. Laryngoscope 2004;114(3):434–9.

[27] Campanini A, De Vito A, Frassineti A, et al. Role of skin-lined tracheotomy in obstructive sleep apnea syndrome: personal experience. Acta Otorhinolaryngol Ital 2004;24(2):68–74.

[28] Kim S, Eisele D, Smith P, et al. Evaluation of patients with sleep apnea after tracheotomy. Arch Otolaryngol Head Neck Surg 1998;124(9):996–1000.

[29] Riley R, Powell N, Li K, et al. Surgery obstructive sleep apnea: long-term clinical outcomes. Otolaryngol Head Neck Surg 2000;112:415–21.

[30] Miller F, Watson D, Malis D. Role of the tongue base suspension suture with the Repose sys-tem bone screw in the multilevel surgical management of obstructive sleep apnea. Otolaryngol Head Neck Surg 2002;126(4):392–8.

[31] Miller F, Watson D, Boseley M. The role of the Genial bone advancement trephine system in

conjunction with uvulopalatopharyngoplasty in the multilevel management of obstructive sleep apnea. Otolaryngol Head Neck Surg 2004;13(1):73–9.

[32] Steward D. Effectiveness of multilevel (tongue and palate) radiofrequency tissue ablation for patients with obstructive sleep apnea syndrome. Laryngoscope 2004;114(12):2073–84.

[33] Stuck B, Starzak K, Hein G, et al. Combined radiofrequency surgery of the tongue base and soft palate in obstructive sleep apnoea. Acta Otolaryngol 2004;124(7):827–32.

[34] Lequeux T, Chantrain G, Bonnand M, et al. Physiotherapy in obstructive sleep apnea syndrome: preliminary results. Eur Arch Otorhinolaryngol, in press.

[35] Spiegel J, Raval T. Overnight hospital stay is not always necessary after uvulopalatopharyngoplasty. Laryngoscope 2005;115(1):167–71.

[36] Mickelson S, Hakim I. Is postoperative intensive care monitoring necessary after uvulopalatopharyngoplasty? Otolaryngol Head Neck Surg 1998;119(4):352–6.

ELSEVIER
SAUNDERS

Anesthesiology Clin N Am
23 (2005) 535–549

ANESTHESIOLOGY
CLINICS OF
NORTH AMERICA

Obstructive Sleep Apnea Syndrome in Children

Preetam Bandla, MD[a,b], Lee J. Brooks, MD[a,b],
Tara Trimarchi, MSN, RN[c], Mark Helfaer, MD, FCCM[b,d],*

[a]*Pulmonary Division, Sleep Disorders Center, Children's Hospital of Philadelphia,
34th Street and Civic Center Boulevard, Philadelphia, PA 19104-4399, USA*
[b]*University of Pennsylvania School of Medicine, 3400 Spruce Street, Philadelphia, PA 19104, USA*
[c]*Pediatric Intensive Care Unit, Children's Hospital of Philadelphia, 34th Street and Civic Center
Boulevard, Philadelphia, PA 19104-4399, USA*
[d]*Critical Care Medicine, Children's Hospital of Philadelphia, 34th Street and Civic Center Boulevard,
Philadelphia, PA 19104-4399, USA*

The obstructive sleep apnea syndrome (OSAS) is characterized by recurrent episodes of partial or complete obstruction of the upper airway during sleep, resulting in the disruption of normal ventilation and sleep patterns [1]. The symptoms, polysomnographic findings, pathophysiology, and treatment of OSAS are significantly different from those seen in adults (Table 1).

OSAS occurs in children of all ages, but it is most common among preschoolers, when adenotonsillar hypertrophy also is most common. The prevalence of OSAS in children is estimated to be approximately 2% and occurs equally among boys and girls [2]. This distribution contrasts with adults, in whom the prevalence is preponderant among men.

Pathophysiology

Obstructive sleep apnea in children occurs as a result of multiple factors, including airway structure and neuromuscular control, and other factors such as hormonal and genetic influences.

* Corresponding author. University of Pennsylvania School of Medicine, 3400 Spruce Street, Philadelphia, PA 19104.
E-mail address: helfaer@email.chop.edu (M. Helfaer).

Table 1
Features of obstructive sleep apnea in children and adults

Features	Children	Adults
Clinical characteristics		
Peak age	Preschool	Middle age
Gender ratio	Equal male and female	Male predominance, postmenopausal females
Causes	Adenotonsillar hypertrophy, obesity, craniofacial abnormalies	Obesity
Body habitus	Failure to thrive, normal, obese	Obesity
Excessive daytime somnolence	Uncommon	Very common
Neurobehavioral	Hyperactivity, developmental delay, cognitive impairment	Cognitive impairment, impaired vigilance
Polysomnographic findings		
Obstructive respiratory events	Cyclic obstruction or prolonged obstructive hypoventilation	Cyclic obstruction
Sleep architecture	Normal	Decreased delta and REM sleep
Sleep state	REM sleep	REM or non-REM
Cortical arousal	≤50% of apneic episodes	At termination of apneic episodes
Treatment	Primarily surgical (adenotonsillectomy) CPAP secondarily	Primarily CPAP, surgery secondarily (uvulopharyngoplasty)

Abbreviation: REM, rapid eye movement.

Airway anatomy

Structural factors play a major role in the pathophysiology of OSAS. Many children with OSAS have some degree of upper-airway narrowing as a result of either one or a combination of the following: adenotonsillar hypertrophy, craniofacial anomalies, or excess adipose tissue resulting from obesity. In otherwise normal children, tonsillectomy and adenoidectomy usually resolve symptoms and normalize polysomnographic findings [3]. Developmental changes occur in laryngeal dimensions in normal children that are exaggerated under the influence of sedation [4].

Obesity and obstructive sleep apnea in children

Obesity is a well-documented risk factor for the development of OSAS in adults. In contrast, children with OSAS often are of normal weight, and some may even experience a failure to thrive [5]. However, obesity has been increasingly recognized as a risk factor for the development of OSAS in the pediatric population [6–8].

In a large epidemiologic study [2] of 399 children and adolescents aged 2 to 18 years, obesity (defined by a body mass index [BMI] ≥28) was the strongest predictor of sleep-disordered breathing, with an odds ratio of 4.59. Approximately one third of obese children have abnormal polysomnographic findings [6]. In another study [9] of 33 children who were referred for the evaluation of obstructive sleep apnea, obesity was the major predictor of the respiratory disturbance index (number of episodes of apnea plus episodes of hypopnea per hour of sleep) and the lowest level of oxyhemoglobin saturation.

Pathophysiology of obstructive sleep apnea syndrome caused by obesity

There are several hypotheses to explain the relationship between obesity and obstructive sleep apnea. Obesity results in the deposition of adipose tissue within the muscles and soft tissues surrounding the upper airway [10]. This fat deposition along with external compression from the neck and jowls results in the narrowing of the upper airway [11]. The increased chest wall and abdominal mass in obese patients result in reduced lung volumes, especially in the recumbent position. In obese individuals, the cephalad displacement of the abdominal contents and the resultant limitation of diaphragmatic movement can result in a restrictive pulmonary defect, which can contribute to hypoxemia through ventilation-perfusion mismatch and hypoventilation [12]. Obesity also may result in increased pharyngeal "floppiness" if adipose tissue contributes to a relative uncoupling of the pharyngeal mucosa from the effects of the upper-airway dilatory muscles.

Neuromotor factors

A number of factors suggest that neuromotor factors also play a role in the development of OSAS: 1) Children with OSAS only experience obstruction while they are asleep and not awake; 2) a small percentage of otherwise normal children continue to have persistent OSAS even after an adenotonsillectomy [3]; 3) some children with OSAS who undergo adenotonsillectomy with a resolution of disease develop a recurrence of OSAS during adolescence [13]; and 4) although adult women have a smaller pharynx than men, the prevalence of OSAS in women is lower, probably because their pharynx is stiffer and therefore less collapsible [14]. Similarly, although normal children have a smaller upper airway than adults do, their airways are less collapsible, and they snore less and have fewer obstructive apneas. This suggests that normal children compensate for a smaller upper airway by an increased ventilatory drive to their upper-airway muscles [15]. Children with OSAS may have reduced, centrally mediated activation of their upper-airway muscles that results in increased collapsibility of the upper airway [16].

Clinical features

The clinical features of OSAS in children include nocturnal symptoms such as snoring, labored breathing, paradoxical respiratory effort, observed apnea, restlessness, sweating, unusual sleep positions (eg, sleeping sitting up, hyperextension of the neck), and enuresis [17]. Daytime symptoms may include mouth breathing, poor school performance, excessive daytime somnolence, morning headaches, fatigue, hyperactivity, aggression, and social withdrawal.

Children with OSAS usually are of normal height and weight, but obesity has been increasingly recognized as a risk factor [6]. The failure to thrive and developmental delay can occur with OSAS [5]. Other physical findings may include mouth breathing, nasal voice quality, retrognathia, or micrognathia. Tonsillar hypertrophy is a common physical finding in children with OSAS, although its absence neither excludes nor confirms the diagnosis [9].

The size of the adenoids has been shown to correlate with the severity of obstructive apneas on polysomnography [9]; however, a large amount of clinical variability is available, so adenoid size alone cannot be used to establish a diagnosis. Rarely, untreated OSAS resulting in pulmonary hypertension may manifest as a loud pulmonary component of the second heart sound.

Complications

Left untreated, OSAS can result in serious morbidity from various adverse sequelae that occur as a result of chronic nocturnal hypoxemia and sleep fragmentation. Growth impairment can occur with OSAS and, in severe cases, may result in the failure to thrive. After an adenotonsillectomy, children with OSAS may experience a growth spurt [18,19]. This growth spurt appears to be the results of decreased caloric expenditure secondary to decreased work of breathing and an increase in the secretion of insulin-like growth factor-I following adenotonsillectomy [18,19].

Cardiovascular complications such as pulmonary hypertension, cor pulmonale, and heart failure used to be common presentations of OSAS in children, but these are now rare. Treatment of the OSAS reverses cor pulmonale. OSAS in children can result in cardiac remodeling and hypertrophy of both the right and left ventricles, although the exact mechanism of left ventricular hypertrophy is unclear [20]. Children with OSAS show dysregulation of systemic blood pressure in the form of a greater mean blood pressure variability during wakefulness than during sleep, a higher night-to-day systolic blood pressure, and smaller nocturnal dipping of the mean blood pressure [21,22]. The degree of blood pressure dysregulation correlates with the severity of the OSAS. Increased blood pressure variability and decreased nocturnal blood pressure dipping have been shown to be associated with end-organ damage and an increased risk for cardiovascular diseases [23,24].

Untreated OSAS may result in neurocognitive deficits, learning problems, behavioral problems, and attention deficit hyperactivity disorder. Gozal [25] demonstrated a high prevalence of sleep-disordered breathing in poorly performing first grade students. Children treated with tonsillectomy and adenoidectomy had significantly improved grades compared with untreated children.

Evaluation

The "gold standard" for diagnosing OSAS is polysomnography. This test can be performed in infants and children of any age and must be scored and interpreted using age-appropriate criteria [1]. Polysomnography can differentiate between primary snoring (ie, snoring not associated with apnea, excessive arousals, or gas exchange abnormalities) and OSAS. Polysomnography also may predict the success of treatment and postoperative complications [3,26,27].

Children have a different pattern of upper-airway obstruction compared with adults and often will desaturate with relatively short apneas. This pattern is caused by a lower functional residual capacity and a higher respiratory rate compared with adults. Therefore, apneas shorter than the 10-second standard in adult polysomnography may be significant in children [1,28]. Similarly, normal children experience fewer respiratory events than do adults. Whereas normal children do not usually have more than one obstructive apnea per hour of sleep, normal young adults may have as many as five apneic episodes. Many children have partial upper-airway obstruction associated with hypercapnia and hypoxemia, rather than discrete obstructive apneas. This pattern has been termed "obstructive hypoventilation" [1] . Although normative data exist for childhood sleep apnea, the degree of polysomnographic abnormalities that produce sequelae is as yet unclear and therefore warrants intervention [29].

Treatment

The majority of children with OSAS show both symptomatic and polysomnographic resolution after a tonsillectomy and adenoidectomy [3]. Even children with associated medical conditions such as Down syndrome [30] or obesity [31] tend to improve after adenotonsillectomy, although additional treatment may sometimes be needed.

In infants and children in whom an adenotonsillectomy is contraindicated or in those patients who continue to be symptomatic after adenotonsillectomy, continuous positive airway pressure (CPAP) delivered through an appropriate nasal mask interface may be used to treat OSAS successfully [32,33]. This therapy can be challenging, especially in very young or developmentally delayed children. Rarely, a tracheostomy may be necessary in very young patients, patients with craniofacial anomalies and neuromuscular syndromes, or patients who cannot tolerate CPAP or bilevel positive airway pressure (BiPAP) following the failure of adenotonsillectomy to resolve symptoms.

Although supplemental oxygen has been shown to improve oxygenation in patients with OSAS, it does not alter the increased work of breathing or sleep fragmentation [34] and, in fact, may prolong apneas by decreasing hypoxic respiratory drive. A few individuals develop a marked rise in their PCO_2 in response to supplemental oxygen [34].

Perioperative management of the child with obstructive sleep apnea

Respiratory compromise is a well-recognized adverse outcome of anesthesia and surgery in children with obstructive OSAS. The perioperative management of the child with OSAS is complicated frequently by underlying craniofacial or airway abnormalities, neurologic disease, and altered nutritional status (obesity or failure to thrive), as well as by cardiac sequelae of OSAS such as pulmonary hypertension and cor pulmonale. Exaggerated hypoventilation in response to the administration of opioid analgesics and sedatives and postobstructive pulmonary edema also may create challenges to perioperative care. Because of the potential for such respiratory problems, all children with a history of OSAS should receive a comprehensive preanesthesia evaluation and intensive intraoperative and postanesthetic monitoring and care focused on the particular needs of the pathophysiology.

Surgery in children with obstructive sleep apnea syndrome

The most common surgical intervention for the treatment of OSAS in children is adenotonsillectomy. Perioperative respiratory compromise in children with OSAS who have undergone adenotonsillectomy includes laryngospasm, apnea, pulmonary edema, pulmonary hypertensive crisis, and pneumonia [26,27, 35,36]. Up to 20% of children with OSAS who undergo urgent adenotonsillectomy may experience such perioperative respiratory complications [35]. Postoperative respiratory distress in children with OSAS often necessitates tracheal reintubation and mechanical ventilation or the use of noninvasive mechanical ventilation such as CPAP.

Occasionally, particularly in patients with severe OSAS [3] or those with craniofacial malformations, adenotonsillectomy is not sufficient to cure the OSAS. In these selected cases, a uvulopalatopharyngoplasty, a tongue reduction, or a craniofacial reconstruction has been used, with varying success. In the severest cases, when CPAP fails and these surgeries cannot provide the relief of the obstruction, a tracheostomy will bypass the obstruction. Regardless of the type of surgical intervention, clinicians caring for children with OSAS during the perioperative experience must consider risk factors for complications, proactively select anesthetic and postoperative management techniques that minimize respiratory deterioration, employ vigilant monitoring practices, and proactively plan for handling acute respiratory failure.

Preanesthesia evaluation

Box 1 lists the risk factors associated with perioperative respiratory complications in children with OSAS. Based on the known risk factors for complications, preanesthesia screening should routinely include a detailed birth and medical history. Growth assessment, a review of systems for recent respiratory

---

Box 1. Pediatric obstructive sleep apnea syndrome: risk factors for respiratory distress after surgery for OSAS

Age less than 3 years
Bleeding
Concurrent respiratory infection
Congenital heart defects
Craniofacial disease
Failure to thrive
History of cor pulmonale
History of premature birth
Neuromuscular disease
Obesity
Other congenital abnormalities or genetic syndrome
Severe obstructive sleep apnea
Throat Pack not removed

Adapted from Sterni LM, Tunkel DE. Obstructive sleep apnea in children: an update. Pediatr Clin North Am 2003;50:427–43.

---

infection, behavioral issues, and school performance should be evaluated. Troublesome behavior often can be addressed by the relief of OSAS [37]. The results of polysomnography also should be reviewed. In patients with severe OSAS or other risk factors, chest radiography, ECG, and possibly echocardiography to evaluate heart function may dictate a higher level of monitoring and postoperative care, depending on the results. Although routine blood gas analysis is not always needed, obtaining a basic metabolic panel to assess for a compensatory metabolic alkalosis in response to chronic hypercarbia may aid identifying prolonged OSAS and establish baseline acid-base balance.

The American Society of Anesthesiologists' (ASA) physical status classification also will help to identify patients with a higher anesthetic risk. In most cases, OSAS is considered a chronic health condition and warrants a classification of ASA II. Children who experience respiratory failure that requires mechanical ventilatory support and those who have severe anatomical malformations of the airway or morbid neurologic disease may be classified as ASA III or IV. Because congenital malformations associated with difficult airways in children also may cause OSAS, special attention should be paid to the potential for difficult airway management in association with this population [38,39]. The Mallampati classification system has not undergone a rigorous validation in children. When surgery for OSAS is performed on children with syndromes associated with difficult airways (Box 2), alternative plans for establishing an airway should be arranged. For example, the ready availability of a laryngeal

---

Box 2. Pediatric syndromes associated with difficult airway management

Achondroplasia
Airway tumors and hemangiomas
Apert's
Beckwith-Wiedemann
Choanal atresia
Cornelia de Lange
Cystic hygromas and teratomas
DiGeorge
Fractured mandible
Goldenhar's
Juvenile rheumatoid arthritis
Mucopolysaccharidosis
Pierre Robin
Smith-Lemli-Opitz
Treacher Collins
Trisomy 21
Turner's

Adapted from Wetzel RC. Anesthesia and perioperative care. In: Behrman RE, Kliegman RM, Jenson HB, editors. Nelson textbook of pediatrics. 17th edition. New York: Elsevier; 2004. p. 354.

---

mask airway and preparation for an emergency tracheostomy with a surgeon in the operating room during induction are wise practices.

The preanesthesia work-up of children with OSAS requires individualized assessments that will assist clinicians to anticipate specialized perioperative needs such as the continued use of mechanical ventilation during the postoperative period, the prevention of gastroesophageal reflux, and the management of neurologic diseases such as seizure activity, which may precipitate apnea. A detailed history of previous anesthetic experiences, including the technique used for endotracheal intubation and response to opioid analgesics for postoperative pain control, are also important for anticipating perioperative issues.

Intraoperative anesthetic plan

Children with OSAS are known to experience the collapse of upper-airway structures and diminished arousal response to elevation in CO_2 during sleep [16].

There are correlates to sleep-disordered breathing and disordered breathing under the effects of general anesthetics [40], so it can be surmised that this population will present with exacerbation of obstructed breathing and apnea when under the affects of anesthesia [41,42]. Because of the increased risk of airway obstruction and apnea in patients with OSAS, the selection of anesthetic technique requires careful consideration.

Anesthesiologists often choose to perform inhalational rather than intravenous induction of anesthesia in children. Inhalational anesthesia results in the dose-dependent relaxation of the genioglossus muscle and may result in airway occlusion [43–45]. Children with OSAS show an exaggeration of the blunted respiratory drive in response to opioid and benzodiazepine administration [41,46] and are at risk for airway obstruction [47]. Waters et al [48] have demonstrated a significant increase in OSAS symptoms in children with OSAS who received a single dose of fentanyl after inhalational anesthetic induction. The researchers reported that 46% of children with known OSAS who continued to breathe spontaneously after receiving an inhaled anesthetic (39% oxygen, 60% nitrous oxide, and 5% halothane mixture) developed complete apnea after a single dose of fentanyl, 0.5 μg/kg. In light of these findings, both inhaled and intravenous anesthesia should be carefully titrated to the effect, particularly when used in combination. Presedation with opioids or benzodiazepines or both before surgery should be used with appropriate preoperative monitoring.

In addition to careful titration of the anesthetic, a neuromuscular blockade for children with OSAS is often used to facilitate endotracheal intubation with an oral RAE endotracheal tube. If the anesthesiologist chooses to avoid a neuromuscular blockade, an adequate depth of anesthesia must be assured to avoid injury resulting from movement when the suspension devices are used by the surgeon. Skilled clinicians and the equipment for managing a difficult airway, such as a fiber-optic laryngoscope as well as a laryngeal mask airway, also should be readily available.

A heightened concern regarding the need to employ difficult airway techniques is particularly prudent in children with OSAS because of craniofacial or known anatomical airway abnormalities. In adult patients with OSAS, the two-person ventilation method (one for holding the jaw position and mask and the other for manual ventilation) and laryngeal mask airway are reported to be helpful for airway management during the induction of anesthesia [38,39,49,50], and are also useful for a minority of children. Of all of the potential maneuvers, the jaw thrust to treat airway obstruction in these patients is the most useful [51] and is superior to the chin lift. Other maneuvers and lateral positioning also are helpful [45]. Antireflux medications and antisialagogue drugs are important adjuncts to consider for the prevention of aspiration and laryngospasm in the OSAS population.

Monitoring anesthesia during surgery in children with OSAS involves a standard approach of continuous electrocardiogram, end-tidal gas, and carbon dioxide concentrations, pulse oximetry and temperature. Rarely, invasive hemodynamic monitoring such as intra-arterial blood pressure measurements are required to manage patients with heart failure, pulmonary hypertension, or severe bronchospasm. The intraoperative assessment of arterial blood gases aids in determining ventilation settings during anesthesia.

Extubating the child with OSAS also is challenging. "Deep extubation" is occasionally practiced but presents some unique challenges because the child with OSAS will be less likely to breath spontaneously and maintain airway patency while under the residual effects of anesthesia. The greatest concern when extubating a child from deep anesthesia is laryngospasm. Many interventions can minimize this complication, including magnesium administration [52] and premedication with midazolam. Desflurane is a less optimal choice than other inhalational agents are when planning a deep extubation [53,54]. When possible, children with OSAS are extubated when they are fully awake and demonstrating markers of airway muscle control such as age-appropriate respiratory rate without assisted ventilation. In addition, adequate muscle strength must be assured before extubation. Extubation should take place in the operating room or in an intensive care unit, where skilled personnel, medications, and equipment required for reintubation are readily available. Occasionally, children with OSAS who do not breathe adequately after surgery can be placed on noninvasive mechanical ventilation, such as mask or nasal CPAP, immediately after extubation [50]. Total intravenous approaches are used rather than inhaled anesthetic techniques, although some of the advantages may not be consistent [55].

Postoperative care

During the postoperative period, all children with OSAS are at risk for respiratory failure because of increased episodes of apnea from baseline, acute airway obstruction, atelectasis, and postobstructive pulmonary edema. Children who have a history of pulmonary hypertension and cor pulmonale also may be at risk for circulatory failure. Because of the risk for serious adverse events, children with severe OSAS or cardiovascular disease or those who are recovering from airway or craniofacial surgery should be monitored after surgery in the pediatric intensive care unit. Most children with mild to moderate OSAS, however, do not require postoperative monitoring in an intensive care unit [56].

Monitoring

The American Academy of Pediatrics recommends postoperative inpatient monitoring for children at high risk for complications associated with OSAS [57]. Depending on the severity of the preoperative cardiopulmonary disturbances, the conduct of the anesthetic, and the physiologic disturbances in the immediate postoperative period, inpatient monitoring should be tailored accordingly. Rarely, patients who do not experience respiratory compromise during the initial recovery phase still may require continued monitoring because obstructive apnea may recur along with the return of REM sleep on postanesthesia day 2 or 3 [43,58]. These patients often are most identified preoperatively by severe sleep-disordered breathing.

Respiratory support

The use of supplemental oxygen during recovery from anesthesia in the child with OSAS is controversial. Administering supplemental oxygen may prolong apnea time and thus prevent the frequency of hypoxemic episodes that are experienced postoperatively. Often, desaturations are a marker for apnea, and these desaturations and apneas may be very common. Even on the first post-operative day, these disturbances may be less severe than those that occurred preoperatively [56]. Hyperoxygenation can mask hypoventilation, making it difficult to determine the severity of postoperative apnea. Children who experience postanesthetic hypoxemia should be evaluated first for pulmonary edema, atelectasis, and pneumonia. If no cause for the hypoxemia other than hypoventilation is identified, the application of noninvasive mechanical ventilation such as CPAP and BiPAP, administered through a facemask, nasal prongs, or a nasal-pharyngeal tube (shortened nasotracheal tube), should be considered in lieu of or in addition to supplemental oxygen. In patients who use noninvasive ventilatory support at baseline or have pulmonary hypertension or who are known to have a markedly depressed respiratory drive, prophylactic postoperative ventilation through an endotracheal tube and ventilator or through a noninvasive means should be considered. Friedman et al [59] have reported success using bilevel nasal CPAP immediately after tonsillectomy and adenoidectomy in children with severe OSAS caused by neuromuscular disease and obesity. Mechanical ventilation can then be discontinued when the child is fully awake and no longer experiencing apnea greater than baseline. Rarely, blood gas analysis that demonstrates baseline values while the patient is spontaneously breathing can guide extubation decisions.

Postobstructive pulmonary edema is an additional respiratory problem in children with OSAS that warrants attention. Postobstructive pulmonary edema occurs because of increased pulmonary blood flow and pulmonary microvascular pressures, which occur as a patient generates an exceedingly high negative inspiratory force while inhaling against a collapsed pharynx or closed glottis [41,50]. Diffuse punctuate hemorrhages are found in the lungs of individuals who experience postobstructive pulmonary edema, suggesting a hemorrhagic nature to the process, as well [60,61]. This phenomenon has been reported previously in children who experienced airway obstruction because of croup and epiglottitis [62,63]. In a more recent study [64] of adult patients with OSAS undergoing tracheostomy, an incidence of postobstructive pulmonary edema as high as 60% has been reported, with the greatest associated morbidity in patients who had cor pulmonale. This clinical situation is rare and poorly understood in children with OSAS. Signs of postobstructive pulmonary edema include hypoxemia, cough, production of serous, frothy or bloody sputum, and crackles in the lung fields on auscultation. Radiographic evidence of alveolar edema, such as diffuse haziness on chest radiography, also will be present. Postobstructive pulmonary edema in the child with OSAS may necessitate reintubation of the trachea and positive pressure mechanical ventilation or noninvasive positive pressure, supplemental oxygen, or the administration of a diuretic.

Pain management

Children with OSAS are known to have a blunted ventilatory response to carbon dioxide, thus opioid analgesics, which will further depress respiratory drive and relax the pharyngeal dilator muscles, must be used judiciously during the postoperative period [46,48]. Whenever possible, opioid-sparing adjuncts, nonopioid analgesics, and nonpharmacologic pain control measures should be used in the postoperative care of children with OSAS. When pain control with moderate to high doses of opioids must be used, prolonged endotracheal intubation and mechanical ventilation may be required. Using opioid analgesia in all cases of OSAS requires that vigilant cardiorespiratory monitoring with continuous pulse oximetry be maintained. With the exception of acetaminophen, nonsteroidal anti-inflammatory drugs have been associated with postoperative bleeding [65] in most studies, although this reaction is controversial [66,67]. Local infiltration of local anesthetic has been studied, with some success at reducing postoperative pain [68–70]. It is clear that aspirin is the poorest choice for postoperative analgesia in this setting because of the prolonged time of action as well as observed increases in hemorrhage. Acetaminophen seems to be the safest choice as either a narcotic-sparing or a primary analgesic, with limited risk of bleeding or airway compromise.

Prognosis

The long-term prognosis and the natural history of childhood OSAS is unknown. It is not known whether children with OSAS will develop OSAS as adults or whether these are two discrete entities. A study by Guilleminault et al [13] has demonstrated a 13% recurrence rate in adolescents who had been successfully treated for childhood OSAS. This suggests that children with OSAS, despite treatment, may be at a higher risk for the development of adult OSAS if they acquire additional risk factors such as androgen secretion at puberty, weight gain, or excessive alcohol ingestion. Most of the complications of OSAS, including cor pulmonale, behavioral problems, and growth impairment, are reversible after successful treatment.

References

[1] American Thoracic Society. Standards and indications for cardiopulmonary sleep studies in children. Am J Respir Crit Care Med 1996;153(2):866–78.

[2] Redline S, Tishler PV, Schluchter M, et al. Risk factors for sleep-disordered breathing in children: associations with obesity, race, and respiratory problems. Am J Respir Crit Care Med 1999;159(5 Pt 1):1527–32.

[3] Suen JS, Arnold JE, Brooks LJ. Adenotonsillectomy for treatment of obstructive sleep apnea in children. Arch Otolaryngol Head Neck Surg 1995;121(5):525–30.

[4] Litman RS, Weissend EE, Shibata D, et al. Developmental changes of laryngeal dimensions in unparalyzed, sedated children. Anesthesiology 2003;98(1):41–5.

[5] Brouillette RT, Fernbach SK, Hunt CE. Obstructive sleep apnea in infants and children. J Pediatr 1982;100(1):31–40.

[6] Marcus CL, Curtis S, Koerner CB, et al. Evaluation of pulmonary function and polysomnography in obese children and adolescents. Pediatr Pulmonol 1996;21(3):176–83.

[7] Mallory Jr GB, Fiser DH, Jackson R. Sleep-associated breathing disorders in morbidly obese children and adolescents. J Pediatr 1989;115(6):892–7.

[8] Silvestri JM, Weese-Mayer DE, Bass MT, et al. Polysomnography in obese children with a history of sleep-associated breathing disorders. Pediatr Pulmonol 1993;16(2):124–9.

[9] Brooks LJ, Stephens BM, Bacevice AM. Adenoid size is related to severity but not the number of episodes of obstructive apnea in children. J Pediatr 1998;132(4):682–6.

[10] Horner RL, Mohiaddan RH, Lowell DG, et al. Sites and sizes of fat deposits around the pharynx in obese patients with obstructive sleep apnoea and weight matched controls. Eur Respir J 1989;2(7):613–22.

[11] Suratt PM, Dee P, Atkinson RL, et al. Fluoroscopic and computed tomographic features of the pharyngeal airway in obstructive sleep apnea. Am Rev Respir Dis 1983;127(4):487–92.

[12] Naimark A, Cherniack RM. Compliance of the respiratory system and its components in health and obesity. J Appl Physiol 1960;15:377–82.

[13] Guilleminault C, Partinen M, Praud JP, et al. Morphometric facial changes and obstructive sleep apnea in adolescents. J Pediatr 1989;114(6):997–9.

[14] Brooks LJ, Strohl KP. Size and mechanical properties of the pharynx in healthy men and women. Am Rev Respir Dis 1992;146:1394–7.

[15] Marcus CL, Fernandes Do Prado LB, Lutz J, et al. Developmental changes in upper airway dynamics. J Appl Physiol 2004;97:98–108.

[16] Marcus CL, Katz ES, Lutz J, et al. Upper airway dynamic responses in children with the obstructive sleep apnea syndrome. Pediatr Res 2005;57(1):99–107.

[17] Brooks LJ, Topol HI. Enuresis in children with sleep apnea. J Pediatr 2003;142(5):515–8.

[18] Marcus CL, Carroll JL, Koerner CB, et al. Determinants of growth in children with the obstructive sleep apnea syndrome. J Pediatr 1994;125(4):556–62.

[19] Bar A, Tarasiuk A, Segev Y, et al. The effect of adenotonsillectomy on serum insulin-like growth factor-I and growth in children with obstructive sleep apnea syndrome. J Pediatr 1999;135(1):76–80.

[20] Amin RS, Kimball TR, Bean JA, et al. Left ventricular hypertrophy and abnormal ventricular geometry in children and adolescents with obstructive sleep apnea. Am J Respir Crit Care Med 2002;165(10):1395–9.

[21] Amin RS, Carroll JL, Jeffries JL, et al. Twenty-four-hour ambulatory blood pressure in children with sleep-disordered breathing. Am J Respir Crit Care Med 2004;169(8):950–6.

[22] Verdecchia P, Schillaci G, Borgioni C, et al. Altered circadian blood pressure profile and prognosis. Blood Press Monit 1997;2(6):347–52.

[23] Verdecchia P, Clement D, Fagard R, et al. Blood pressure monitoring: task force III: target-organ damage, morbidity and mortality. Blood Press Monit 1999;4(6):303–17.

[24] Sega R, Corrao G, Bombelli M, et al. Blood pressure variability and organ damage in a general population: results from the PAMELA study (Pressioni Arteriose Monitorate E Loro Associazioni). Hypertension 2002;39(2 Pt 2):710–4.

[25] Gozal D. Sleep-disordered breathing and school performance in children. Pediatrics 1998; 102(3 Pt 1):616–20.

[26] Rosen GM, Muckle RP, Mahowald MW, et al. Postoperative respiratory compromise in children with obstructive sleep apnea syndrome: can it be anticipated? Pediatrics 1994;93(5):784–8.

[27] McColley SA, April MM, Carroll JL, et al. Respiratory compromise after adenotonsillectomy in children with obstructive sleep apnea. Arch Otolaryngol Head Neck Surg 1992;118(9):940–3.

[28] American Thoracic Society, Medical Section of the American Lung Association. Indications and standards for cardiopulmonary sleep studies. Am Rev Respir Dis 1989;139(2):559–68.

[29] American Thoracic Society. Cardiorespiratory sleep studies in children: establishment of normative data and polysomnographic predictors of morbidity. Am J Respir Crit Care Med 1999; 160(4):1381–7.

[30] Marcus CL, Keens TG, Bautista DB, et al. Obstructive sleep apnea in children with Down syndrome. Pediatrics 1991;88(1):132–9.

[31] Kudoh F, Sanai A. Effect of tonsillectomy and adenoidectomy on obese children with sleep-associated breathing disorders. Acta Otolaryngol Suppl 1996;523:216–8.

[32] Waters KA, Everett FM, Bruderer JW, et al. Obstructive sleep apnea: the use of nasal CPAP in 80 children. Am J Respir Crit Care Med 1995;152(2):780–5.

[33] Marcus CL, Ward SL, Mallory GB, et al. Use of nasal continuous positive airway pressure as treatment of childhood obstructive sleep apnea. J Pediatr 1995;127(1):88–94.

[34] Marcus CL, Carroll JL, Bamford O, et al. Supplemental oxygen during sleep in children with sleep-disordered breathing. Am J Respir Crit Care Med 1995;152(4 Pt 1):1297–301.

[35] Biavati MJ, Manning SC, Phillips DL. Predictive Factors for respiratory complications after tonsillectomy and adenoidectomy in children. Arch Otolaryngol Head Neck Surg 1997;123: 517–21.

[36] Wilson K, Lakheeram I, Morielli A, et al. Can assessment for obstructive sleep apnea help predict postadenotonsillectomy respiratory complications? Anesthesiology 2002;96:313–22.

[37] Tran KD, Nguyen CD, Weedon J, et al. Child behavior and quality of life in pediatric obstructive sleep apnea. Arch Otolaryngol Head Neck Surg 2005;131(1):52–7.

[38] Benumof JL. Management of the difficult airway. Anesthesiology 1991;75:1087–110.

[39] Benumof JL. Laryngeal mask airway and the ASA difficult airway algorithm. Anesthesiology 1996;84:686–99.

[40] Eastwood PR, Szollosi I, Platt PR, et al. Comparison of upper airway collapse during general anaesthesia and sleep. Lancet 2002;359(9313):1207–9.

[41] Blum RH, McGowan FX. Chronic airway obstruction and cardiac dysfunction: anatomy, pathophysiology and anesthetic implications. Paediatr Anaesth 2004;14:75–83.

[42] Isono S, Shimada A, Utsungi M, et al. Comparison of static mechanical properties of the passive pharynx between normal children and children with sleep-disordered breathing. Am J Respir Crit Care Med 1998;157:1323–7.

[43] Helfaer MA, Wilson MD. Obstructive sleep apnea, control of ventilation and anesthesia in children. Paediatr Anaesth 1994;41:131–51.

[44] Ochiai R, Guthrie RD, Motoyama FK. Differential sensitivity to halothane anesthesia of the genioglossus, intercostals and diaphragm in kittens. Anesth Analg 1992;74:338–44.

[45] Litman RS, Kottra JA, Gallagher PR, et al. Diagnosis of anesthetic-induced upper airway obstruction in children using respiratory inductance plethysmography. J Clin Monit Comput 2002;17(5):279–85.

[46] Strauss SG, Lynn AM, Bratten SL, et al. Ventilatory response to CO_2 in children with obstructive sleep apnea from adenotonsillar hypertrophy. Anesth Analg 1999;89:328–32.

[47] Litman RS, Kottra JA, Berkowitz RJ, et al. Upper airway obstruction during midazolam/nitrous oxide sedation in children with enlarged tonsils. Pediatr Dent 1998;20(5):318–20.

[48] Waters KA, McBrien F, Stewart P. Effects of OSA, inhalational anesthesia and fentanyl on the airway ventilation in children. J Appl Physiol 2002;92:1987–94.

[49] Biro P, Kaplan V, Bloch KE. Anesthetic management of a patient with obstructive sleep apnea syndrome and difficult airway access. J Clin Anesth 1995;7:417–21.

[50] Sterni LM, Tunkel DE. Obstructive sleep apnea in children: an update. Pediatr Clin North Am 2003;50:427–43.

[51] Arai YC, Fukunaga K, Hirota S, et al. The effects of chin lift and jaw thrust while in the lateral position on stridor score in anesthetized children with adenotonsillar hypertrophy. Anesth Analg 2004;99(6):1638–41 [table of contents].

[52] Gulhas N, Durmus M, Demirbilek S, et al. The use of magnesium to prevent laryngospasm after tonsillectomy and adenoidectomy: a preliminary study. Paediatr Anaesth 2003;13(1):43–7.

[53] Valley RD, Freid EB, Bailey AG, et al. Tracheal extubation of deeply anesthetized pediatric patients: a comparison of desflurane and sevoflurane. Anesth Analg 2003;96(5):1320–4.

[54] Wetzel RC. Anesthesia and perioperative care. In: Behrman RE, Kliegman RM, Jenson HB, editors. Nelson textbook of pediatrics. 17th edition. New York: Elsevier; 2004. p. 342–57.

[55] Cohen IT, Drewsen S, Hannallah RS. Propofol or midazolam do not reduce the incidence of emergence agitation associated with desflurane anaesthesia in children undergoing adenotonsillectomy. Paediatr Anaesth 2002;12(7):604–9.

[56] Helfaer MA, McColley SA, Pyzik PL, et al. Polysomnography after adenotonsillectomy in mild pediatric obstructive sleep apnea. Crit Care Med 24(8):1323–7.

[57] AAP Section on Pediatric Pulmonology, Subcommittee on Obstructive Sleep Apnea Syndrome. Clinical practice guidelines: diagnosis and management of childhood obstructive sleep apnea syndrome. Pediatrics 2002;109:704–12.

[58] Reeder MK, Goldman MD, Loh L, et al. Late postoperative nocturnal dips in oxygen saturation in patients undergoing major abdominal vascular surgery: predictive value of pre-operative overnight pulse oximetry. Anesthesia 1992;47:110–5.

[59] Friedman O, Chidekel A, Lawless ST, et al. Postoperative bilevel airway pressure ventilation after tonsillectomy and adenoidectomy in children: a preliminary report. Int J Pediatr Otorhinolaryngol 1999;51:177–80.

[60] Koch SM, Abramson DC, Ford M, et al. Bronchoscopic findings in postobstructive pulmonary oedema. Can J Anaesth 1996;43:73–6.

[61] McConkey PP. Postobstructive pulmonary oedema: a case series and review. Anaesth Intensive Care 2000;28:72–6.

[62] Sofer S, Bar-Ziv J, Scharf SM. Pulmonary edema following relief of upper airway obstruction. Chest 1984;86:401–3.

[63] Galvis AG, Stool SE, Bluestone CD. Pulmonary edema following relief of upper airway obstruction. Ann Otol Rhinol Laryngol 1980;89:124–8.

[64] Burke AJ, Duke SG, Clyne S, et al. Incidence of pulmonary edema after tracheotomy for obstructive sleep apnea. Otolaryngol Head Neck Surg 2001;125:319–23.

[65] Marret E, Flahault A, Samama CM, et al. Effects of postoperative, nonsteroidal, anti-inflammatory drugs on bleeding risk after tonsillectomy: meta-analysis of randomized, controlled trials. Anesthesiology 2003;98(6):1497–502.

[66] Krishna S, Hughes LF, Lin SY. Postoperative hemorrhage with nonsteroidal anti-inflammatory drug use after tonsillectomy: a meta-analysis. Arch Otolaryngol Head Neck Surg 2003;129(10): 1086–9.

[67] Dsida R, Cote CJ. Nonsteroidal anti-inflammatory drugs and hemorrhage following tonsillectomy: do we have the data? Anesthesiology 2004;100(3):749–51.

[68] Goldsher M, Podoshin L, Fradis M, et al. Effects of peritonsillar infiltration on posttonsillectomy pain: a double-blind study. Ann Otol Rhinol Laryngol 1996;105(11):868.

[69] Meoli AL, Rosen CL, Kristo D. Upper airway management of the adult patient with obstructive sleep apnea in the perioperative period: avoiding complications. Sleep 2003;26:1060–5.

[70] Bruppacher H, Reber A, Keller JP, et al. The effects of common airway maneuvers on airway pressure and flow in children undergoing adenoidectomies. Anesth Analg 2003;97(1):29–34.

ELSEVIER
SAUNDERS

Anesthesiology Clin N Am
23 (2005) 551–564

ANESTHESIOLOGY
CLINICS OF
NORTH AMERICA

The Rapid Sequence Induction Revisited: Obesity and Sleep Apnea Syndrome

Eugene B. Freid, MD, FCCM[a,b,*]

[a]Department of Anesthesiology, Nemours Children's Clinics, 807 Children's Way,
Jacksonville, FL 32207, USA
[b]Departments of Anesthesiology and Pediatrics, University of North Carolina School of Medicine,
Chapel Hill, NC 27599-7010, USA

The loss of protective airway reflexes during the induction of general anesthesia can result in pulmonary aspiration of the gastric contents. Pulmonary aspiration remains an infrequent but serious cause of anesthesia-related morbidity and mortality, with little change in incidence over the past 20 years. In a study of 133 cases of aspiration reported to the Australian Anesthetic Incident Monitoring Study database [1], 56% of the cases of pulmonary aspiration occurred during the induction of anesthesia, and obese patients were over-represented in the group of patients who aspirated. Obesity is one of a number of factors that contributes to the risk of aspiration during anesthesia, including emergency surgery, trauma, airway difficulties, inadequate depth of anesthesia, and gastrointestinal disorders such as intestinal obstruction, hiatal hernia, and gastroesophageal reflux.

The technique of rapid sequence induction includes four separate actions designed to reduce the risk of pulmonary aspiration: the use of pharmacologic agents with or without gastric suctioning to reduce gastric acid volume and acidity; the administration of a rapidly acting hypnotic agent and muscle relaxant to limit the apneic time and reduce the at-risk period of an unprotected airway; the application of cricoid pressure; and the absence of mask ventilation after a period of preoxygenation. Although these actions seem simple and logical and are based on basic and clinical science, not one randomized controlled trial has confirmed the benefits of rapid sequence induction. Yet, rapid sequence induction

---

* Department of Anesthesiology, Nemours Children's Clinics, 807 Children's Way, Jacksonville, FL 32207.
  E-mail address: efreid@aims.unc.edu

0889-8537/05/$ – see front matter © 2005 Elsevier Inc. All rights reserved.
doi:10.1016/j.atc.2005.03.010   *anesthesiology.theclinics.com*

is considered the standard of care in US anesthesia practice for all patients with an increased risk of pulmonary aspiration.

The use of rapid sequence induction is common practice in patients with obesity and sleep apnea syndrome. However, aspects of the rapid sequence induction technique may be deleterious in some patients with these disorders. A review of the current medical literature elicits as many questions as answers regarding the usefulness of this technique. This article addresses a number of these questions: Are patients with obesity and sleep apnea really more at risk than the general population for pulmonary gastric aspiration? Does rapid sequence induction reduce the risk of pulmonary acid aspiration? Are there situations in which the rapid sequence induction technique is potentially dangerous in patients with morbid obesity or obstructive sleep apnea? Is cricoid pressure a beneficial technique, and when is it deleterious? Which muscle relaxant and sedative combination is the most useful for rapid sequence induction?

Rapid sequence induction and the difficult airway

The specific alterations in airway anatomy and physiology leading to difficult mask ventilation and tracheal intubation in patients with morbid obesity and sleep apnea syndrome are addressed elsewhere in this issue. A number of important differences in cardiopulmonary physiology that affect the safety of anesthetic induction in these patients also are addressed elsewhere. These anatomic and physiologic differences must be taken into account when considering the risks and benefits of the rapid sequence induction technique in these patients.

Although there are several studies that have concluded that no increased risk of difficult intubation is posed in the morbidly obese population [2,3], numerous other studies demonstrate a clearly defined increased risk of difficult intubation in both the morbidly obese [4–6] and sleep apnea syndrome populations [7–9]. Hiremath et al [10] found that eight of 15 individuals with Cormack and Lehane grade 4 laryngoscopic views had apnea-hypopnea indices consistent with previously undiagnosed sleep apnea syndrome, whereas only two matched controls without a difficult laryngoscopic view had similar scores. Although these data do not establish that patients with sleep apnea syndrome have difficult airways, the authors propose that the two conditions appear to be related and to share anatomic features that act to reduce the skeletal confines of the tongue. Additionally, the incidence of diabetes mellitus is increased in the obese population, and long-standing diabetes mellitus has been associated with an increased risk of difficult intubation caused by the glycosylation of collagen and its deposition in the joints, resulting in limited joint mobility syndrome [11].

The presence of a potentially difficult airway during the induction of anesthesia in obese and sleep apnea syndrome patients is a risk to several aspects of patient safety. The ability to assure oxygenation and ventilation during management of the difficult airway is the paramount concern. A secondary concern is that both difficult airways and the development of inadequate anesthetic depth during difficult airway management have been found to predispose to regurgitation, vomiting, and aspiration, as reported in the Australian Anesthetic Incident Monitoring Study database [1] and in nearly one-third of the patients who aspirated during induction of anesthesia in a study of pulmonary aspiration by Warner et al [12].

Several of the crucial components of the rapid sequence induction technique have even been shown to be deleterious in patients who have potentially difficult airways. A key element in the rapid sequence technique is the nonhypoxemic apneic period, designed to avoid gastric insufflation that would reduce barrier pressure and promote regurgitation. Because the ability to mask ventilate is not tested before the administration of the muscle relaxant, a distinct risk is the development of a cannot-intubate and cannot-ventilate situation. Furthermore, because the functional residual capacity of obese patients is reduced, they develop oxygen desaturation faster than the nonobese, and the safe apneic period is reduced from more than 5 minutes to less than 2 to 3 minutes in the preoxygenated state [13–15]. The absence of ventilation in the rapid sequence technique promotes atelectasis that additionally reduces the apneic duration of adequate oxygenation. A recent study [16] in morbidly obese individuals (limited to 160 kg by the weight limit of the CT scanner) has demonstrated that the administration of constant positive airway pressure (CPAP) during the preoxygenation period and gentle ventilation with positive end-expiratory pressure (PEEP) during anesthetic induction significantly reduce atelectasis, as documented by chest CT scans. An associated benefit to the reduced atelectasis was a significantly increased average PaO_2 (457 ± 130 pascals [Pa] versus 315 ± 100 Pa, $P=0.035$) in those subjects who received CPAP-PEEP versus the control subjects. Theoretically, that increase in PaO_2 would increase the apneic time to oxygen desaturation if an airway event were to occur.

A second component used in the rapid sequence induction that may be deleterious in patients with obesity and sleep apnea syndrome is the use and misuse of cricoid pressure. As discussed later, the correct application of cricoid pressure is difficult for the untrained practitioner and difficult to maintain even for the trained practitioner, and the pressure can affect both the ability to mask ventilate and the direct laryngoscopic view. Allman [17] has demonstrated that the application of cricoid pressure by an experienced anesthetist causes both a significant reduction in mean exhaled tidal volume ($P \leq 0.001$) and an increase in peak inspiratory pressures ($P \leq 0.001$), with complete airway occlusion occurring between 6% and 11% of the time when cricoid pressure is applied. Saghaei and Masoodifar [18] prospectively bimanually applied 4.5 kg (40–50 Newtons [N]) of cricoid force to 80 American Society of Anesthesiologists grade-1 adult patients who were randomly divided into those who received cricoid pressure and controls (simple placement of hands without exerting pressure). The effects on mask ventilation were identical to those of Allman [17], with a significant increase in peak inspiratory pressure and a significant decrease in tidal volume after the application of cricoid pressure ($P \leq 0.001$). Hartsilver and Vanner [19] studied 52 female patients undergoing elective surgery, and facemask ventilation was assessed under five different conditions: no cricoid pressure; backward cricoid pressure applied with a force of 30 N; cricoid pressure applied in an upward and backward direction with a force of 30 N; backward cricoid pressure with a force of 44 N; and cricoid pressure applied with a tracheal tube inserted. The authors found that cricoid pressure applied with a force of 44 N can cause airway obstruction, but if cricoid force is reduced to 30 N, airway obstruction occurs less frequently ($P = 0.0001$), unless the force is applied in an upward and backward direction.

Cricoid pressure can also adversely affect direct laryngoscopy. Haslam et al [20] recorded the laryngoscopic view using a rigid, zero-degree endoscope to define the effect of cricoid pressure on laryngoscopy. In 40 patients undergoing elective surgery, cricoid pressure was increased by 10 N increments, and the change in laryngoscopic view with increasing cricoid pressure was evaluated (Fig. 1). In five subjects in whom the initial laryngoscopic view was good, a marked deterioration in view occurred as cricoid pressure increased. In three of these subjects, the view decreased to completely obscure the larynx at a force of 30, 40, and 60 N, respectively. The laryngeal view was obscured by a down-folding of the epiglottis, adduction of the vestibular folds, and encroachment of the pharyngeal soft tissues into the line of sight, or rotation of the larynx also behind the right aryepiglottic fold during cricoid pressure application.

Because of the potential for airway deformation with cricoid pressure, using the minimum force necessary to prevent gastric regurgitation will optimize the maintenance of a patent airway and an adequate laryngeal view. In patients in whom the laryngoscopic view of the glottis is poor, posteriorly applied cricoid pressure may cause the view to further deteriorate, and although backward and upward laryngeal displacement can improve laryngeal visualization, this displacement unfortunately worsens the ability to mask ventilate. Currently, far more

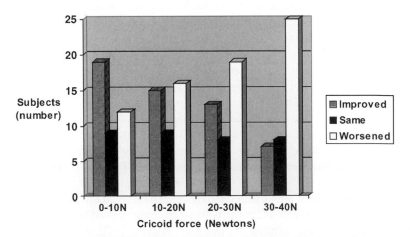

Fig. 1. The number of subjects in whom the laryngoscopic view improved, remained unchanged, or worsened with each 10 N of increase in cricoid force. (*Data from* Haslam N, Parker L, Duggan JE. Effect of cricoid pressure on the view at laryngoscopy. Anaesthesia 2005;60(1):41–7.)

morbidity occurs owing to hypoxemia during difficult or failed intubation than from aspiration. If the need to mask ventilate is crucial, the cricoid pressure should be directed directly posterior and may need to be gradually released.

Failed intubation in rapid sequence induction is an uncommon event, even in patients with morbid obesity. The incidence of failed intubation in the general population is approximately 1:2300 in the general population and 1:230 in the obstetric population [21,22]. In a 1999 survey of academic anesthetists in the United Kingdom, 94 of 209 respondents (45%) had experienced failed intubation during rapid sequence induction at least once in their career [23]. The incidence of failed intubation in the morbidly obese population is ill defined. In the study of difficult intubation in morbid obesity by Juvin et al [6], there were no cases of failed intubation, but as many as eight attempts at direct laryngoscopy by as many as four persons were required. Brodsky et al [3] had one failed rapid sequence induction in 100 subjects with a body mass index (BMI) greater than 40 kg/m^2. In a study of 117 morbidly obese parturients whose weight exceeded 136.4 kg (300 pounds) at the time of delivery, general anesthesia was administered to 17 patients. Difficult tracheal intubation occurred in six of the 17 morbidly obese parturients, compared with zero of eight nonobese control subjects ($P = 0.06$). There were no failed intubations, but two of the morbidly obese patients underwent an awake laryngoscopy or intubation [24].

Unfortunately, several of the techniques commonly used in the failed intubation algorithm also may be adversely affected by cricoid pressure. Cricoid pressure has been shown to make laryngeal mask airway (LMA) insertion more difficult [25,26] and makes the use of the intubating LMA less likely to be successful [27]. Because of these potentially adverse affects of cricoid pressure on ventilation, laryngoscopy, and laryngeal mask insertion, most failed intubation guidelines now recommend placing the patient in Trendelenburg position, with suction available and graded release of cricoid pressure in the cannot-intubate, cannot-ventilate situation.

Risk of gastroesophageal reflux and pulmonary aspiration

In common practice, obese patients are considered a group that is at increased risk for gastric aspiration, but what are the supporting data that all obese patients are at a higher risk of gastric acid aspiration? Because the use of rapid sequence induction has not been proven to prevent gastric aspiration and may be hazardous in some circumstances, is it reasonable to apply the technique to all obese individuals? Factors that increase the risk for pulmonary gastric aspiration syndrome include low pH of the gastric contents; an increased volume of gastric fluid, which depends on both the production of gastric fluid and on gastric emptying; the presence of gastroesophageal reflux, which depends on the barrier pressure between the stomach and lower esophageal sphincter; and the time fasted. A number of authors have evaluated the risk of gastroesophageal reflux in the morbidly obese patient. Several authors have demonstrated a rate of gastroesophageal reflux similar to the general population. Warner et al [12] found no increase in the incidence of aspiration in those with a body mass index greater than 35 kg/ m². Zacchi et al [28] demonstrated a resistance gradient between the stomach and gastroesophageal junction comparable to nonobese individuals. Kadar et al [29] reported 650 mask general anesthetics for electroconvulsive therapy in 50 obese subjects with no episodes of clinical pulmonary aspiration, although asymptomatic reflux or aspiration may have been present. Coussa et al [16] found no evidence of gastric aspiration on the chest CT scans of 18 morbidly obese subjects after anesthetic induction without cricoid pressure, including nine patients who received gentle mechanical ventilation with PEEP by mask.

Recently, several studies have demonstrated an increased risk of reflux in the morbidly obese [30,31]. Fisher et al [30] reported 30 subjects with morbid obesity presenting for bariatric surgery evaluation. Sixteen of the 30 patients had symptomatic reflux, and 11 of the 30 had abnormal esophageal acid exposure (pH ≤ 4 for more than 5% of observed time) as determined by pH probe and esophageal manometry. Individuals with abnormal acid exposure had a body mass index that was larger than were those without abnormal acid exposure (BMI of 56.5 versus 48.3 kg/m², $P \leq 0.05$), even though lower esophageal sphincter pressure was not correlated with body mass index. In addition to the baseline risk of gastroesophageal reflux, obese individuals also are more likely to have diabetes mellitus and be prone to gastroparesis.

There are conflicting data regarding the risk of gastroesophageal reflux specifically in patients with obstructive sleep apnea. Because the transdiaphragmatic pressure increases in parallel with the increased intrathoracic pressure generated during obstructive apnea episodes, the attendant increases in gastric volume and pressure can lead to passive regurgitation whenever there is lower esophageal sphincter insufficiency [32]. On the other hand, there are data showing that sleep apnea syndrome and gastroesophageal reflux are common entities that share similar risk factors but appear not to be linked causally [33].

Cricoid pressure

Cricoid pressure provides a second line of defense when the lower esophageal sphincter fails to prevent passive regurgitation. The practice of cricoid pressure is attributed to Sellick [34] in 1961, but its use to obstruct the esophagus is over 200 years old. Monro [35] in the 1770s, Hunter in 1776 [35], and Curry in 1796 [36] described the use of esophageal compression at the throat to assist ventilation and reduce gastric insufflation during resuscitation.

The original study by Sellick postdated by 10 years the description by Morton and Wylie [37] of protecting the airway with the patient in the sitting position using barbiturate and relaxant, followed by rapid intubation. When evaluating the data reported by Sellick [34], it is essential to remember that his technique was different from cricoid pressure as practiced today. In that study, cricoid pressure prevented fluid passing from esophagus under the cricoid ring and at lower pressures controlled the flow of fluid. The patient's head was extended as if for a tonsillectomy rather than in the "sniffing" position to increase the anterior convexity of the cervical spine, thus stretching the esophagus to prevent lateral displacement. Unfortunately this position also makes laryngoscopy more difficult, and most patients undergoing anesthetic induction are in the sniffing rather than extended neck position. Sellick also used a light Trendelenburg position to help clear any leakage away from airway. He then evaluated 26 high-risk patients using cricoid pressure. None of the patients demonstrated reflux during the application of the cricoid pressure, and three had reflux subsequently, after cricoid pressure was released, supporting the effectiveness of the technique.

Despite considerable dogma regarding the benefits of cricoid pressure in the past 40 years, the use of cricoid pressure is being revisited as recent information supports a reevaluation of the use of this seemingly simple and safe technique. Unfortunately, a well-designed controlled, randomized prospective trial of cricoid pressure has not been performed. Brimacombe and Berry [38], Ng and Smith [39], and Landsman [40] have examined the topic of cricoid pressure and provided comprehensive reviews describing the advantages and risks associated with the technique. Some authors have described the technique as cricoid force rather than pressure because the downward force is measured in Newtons rather than in millimeters of mercury (30 N of cricoid pressure is equivalent to 40 mm Hg of upper esophageal sphincter pressure).

There are unquestionably data to support the practice of cricoid pressure. In the study by Sellick [34], the reflux of gastric contents occurred in three of 26 patients when cricoid pressure was released. A 30-N cricoid force provided protection against gastric reflux even with 40 mm Hg of upper esophageal sphincter pressure in cadavers with the head extended [41]. A 40-N cricoid force increased the upper esophageal sphincter pressure to more than 38 mm Hg in 24 patients, with or without a pillow under their head [42]. Also, cricoid pressure has been shown to prevent gastric insufflation in both adults [43] and children [44,45] during mask ventilation.

Data are also evolving against the routine use of cricoid pressure. As discussed above, cricoid pressure can impede airway patency and make direct laryngoscopy more difficult, clearly vital issues during the induction of anesthesia in those with obesity and sleep apnea syndrome. It is important to remember that airway difficulty itself has been demonstrated to be an independent factor in pulmonary aspiration [12].

Second, cricoid pressure has been demonstrated to reduce lower esophageal pressure by a yet uncertain mechanism. The lower esophageal pressure, which is normally 25 to 35 mmHg, is the first line of defense against the passive regurgitation of gastric contents. Lower esophageal sphincter pressure falls with most anesthetic induction and nondepolarizing neuromuscular blocking agents, reducing the barrier pressure (lower esophageal pressure minus gastric pressure). Intragastric pressure is normally less than 7 mm Hg at rest, but succinylcholine increases intragastric pressure to 40 mm Hg, and during vomiting, intragastric pressure rises to 45 mm Hg. Tournadre et al [46] studied eight healthy, fasted awake volunteers who underwent intragastric, esophageal, and lower esophageal sphincter (LES) pressure monitoring. Cricoid pressures of 20 N followed by 40 N were each applied for 15 seconds. The application of cricoid pressure reduced LES pressure from 24 ± 3 to 15 ± 4 mm Hg at a force of 20 N ($P \leq 0.05$) and to 12 ± 4 mm Hg with a force of 40 N ($P \leq 0.01$). Garrard et al [47] reported a similar reduction in lower esophageal sphincter pressure during the application of cricoid pressure in anaesthetized patients. The gastric pressure was less than the esophageal pressure, and the barrier to reflux remained intact in all cases.

If cricoid pressure were universally beneficial, there would be few cases of pulmonary aspiration when cricoid pressure was used and, alternatively, many cases when cricoid pressure and rapid sequence induction were not used. In the Australian Anesthetic Incident Monitoring Study [1], 11 patients (8% of those with pulmonary aspiration) experienced aspiration despite the application of cricoid pressure. Warner et al [12] retrospectively reviewed the perioperative courses of 172,334 consecutive patients 18 years of age or older who underwent 215,488 general anesthetic procedures from July 1985 to June 1991 and found pulmonary aspiration had occurred in 67 patients. Of the 67 patients who aspirated, 33 did so during induction, and 14 patients had pulmonary aspiration despite rapid sequence induction. In a survey exploring anesthetists' practice in rapid sequence induction in the United Kingdom, 59 of 209 respondents (28%) had seen regurgitation with rapid sequence induction, and three respondents reported the death of a patient as a result of regurgitation with rapid sequence induction [23]. In a prospective study from France, at a time when cricoid pressure was rarely used, there was a lower rate of aspiration during anesthesia than in comparable studies in countries where cricoid pressure was used [48].

Another problem with the use of cricoid pressure is that cricoid pressure is often incorrectly or inconsistently applied in the clinical setting [49]. Untrained individuals do not apply the correct amount of force, and it is often not sustained for the entire duration that the airway is unprotected [50]. It has been suggested that training in the application of cricoid pressure or the use of a mechanical device be used to assure correct and consistent application of the cricoid pressure.

Even when cricoid pressure is correctly applied, there is no guarantee that the esophagus will be actually occluded between the posterior cricoid ring and the vertebral body. In a recent study [51], 22 awake healthy volunteers underwent sagittal and axial magnetic resonance imaging of their necks, with their heads in a neutral position at baseline and with 20 to 30 N of applied cricoid force. In 53% of the patients at baseline, the esophagus was viewed lateral to the cricoid ring, and in 90% of the subjects, the esophagus was found to be displaced laterally after cricoid pressure was applied (Fig. 2). Lateral laryngeal displacement was noted in 67% of the subjects with cricoid pressure, and airway compression of at least 1 mm was demonstrated in 81% of the subjects as a result of cricoid pressure. The authors, based on their results, challenged the assumption that the cricoid, esophagus, and vertebral body are juxtaposed along the axial plane.

In addition to airway compromise, there are other complications of cricoid pressure, both common and unusual. The timing of the application of cricoid

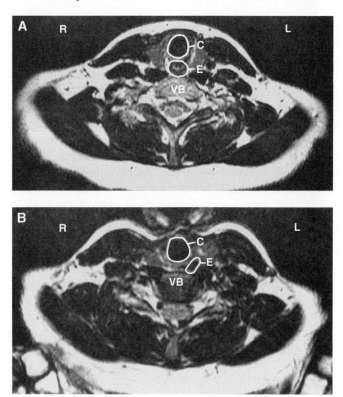

Fig. 2. The esophagus is seen at midline before cricoid pressure (*A*) and is deviated laterally with cricoid pressure (*B*). Note that the esophagus is only partially occluded. C, cricoid; E, esophagus; VB, vertebral body. (*From* Smith KJ, Dobranowski J, Yip G, et al. Cricoid pressure displaces the esophagus: an observational study using magnetic resonance imaging. Anesthesiology 2003;99:60–4. with permission.)

pressure is critical. If it is applied before the loss of consciousness or with too much force, it is painful and may lead to vomiting or retching, which could promote pulmonary aspiration. Before the loss of consciousness, the currently used force of 30 to 40 N is too uncomfortable for volunteers to tolerate. Awake volunteers tolerated 20 N of cricoid force, whereas 40 N caused difficulty in breathing in 50% of volunteers [52]. Cricoid pressure also can have a negative hemodynamic consequence. Saghaei and Masoodifar [18] found a mean 20-mm Hg increase in systolic arterial blood pressure ($P \leq 0.001$) and a mean 10-beat per minute increase in heart rate ($P \leq 0.001$) occurred as a result of the application of 45 N of cricoid pressure in healthy adult patients after induction of anesthesia with sodium thiopental, 5 mg/kg, fentanyl, 1 μg/kg, and 1% halothane by mask. Rare complications of cricoid pressure have been described, including esophageal rupture, which can occur during active vomiting. Cricoid pressure should be released during active vomiting. Data suggest that a nasogastric tube does not impair the efficacy of cricoid pressure. Studies support suctioning the nasogastric tube before induction and leaving the nasogastric tube open to allow the intra-gastric pressure to be released [53].

The optimal cricoid force that will provide a barrier to reflux yet minimize airway and respiratory compromise has been recently reappraised as well. The force believed initially to be required to provide a barrier to reflux was 40 N and was subsequently reduced to 30 N. Recent data suggest that 20 N may be suffi-cient to provide the second layer of protection at the upper esophageal sphincter yet minimize the distortion of the airway. Haslam et al [54] studied the gastric pressure in a large group of heterogeneous surgical patients during rapid se-quence induction with sodium thiopental and succinylcholine. The highest gastric pressure observed was 14 mm Hg, and most values were considerably less than this value. This demonstrates a gastric barrier pressure of less than 15 mm Hg, even with wide-open gastroesophageal reflux under these conditions. The authors have concluded that cricoid pressure applied at 20 N of force is more than adequate to protect most anesthetized patients from regurgitation. Until more data confirm the low gastric pressure, the current recommendations are to initiate cricoid pressure with a force of 20 N as the induction agents are administered and to increase the force to 30 N as loss of consciousness occurs.

Does induction agent pharmacology make a difference?

Historically, succinylcholine is the neuromuscular blocking agent of choice in rapid sequence induction, for numerous reasons. It has the most rapid onset and shortest duration of action of currently available neuromuscular blocking drugs. The rapid onset is essential to reduce the apneic period and shorten the at-risk period with an unprotected airway. The short duration of action is critical if the airway is difficult and it is required for the patient to resume spontaneous ventilation. Several authors have suggested recently that reducing the dose of succinylcholine to 0.6 mg/kg still allows adequate intubation conditions, and the lower dose would be attractive as far as reducing the time to return to spon-taneous ventilation [55,56]. However, it should be remembered that inadequate anesthetic depth and incomplete muscle relaxation are independent variables that lead to pulmonary aspiration [1,12].

Unfortunately, succinylcholine has a number of well-described side effects. One side effect that affects the risk of aspiration itself during rapid sequence induction is fasciculations that cause a rise in gastric pressure [57]. Succinylcho-line has been demonstrated to increase the gastric pressure to 40 mm Hg, al-though recent reports do not demonstrate this degree of gastric pressure increase [54]. The practice of defasciculation will restrict the intragastric pressure rise but will require that a larger dose of succinylcholine be administered. Brodsky and Foster [58] have reported data from 14 morbidly obese patients who received succinylcholine without pretreatment with a nondepolarizing blocking agent. Only three of the 14 patients had gross fasciculations, and only two of the 14 individuals developed myalgia, suggesting that the morbidly obese do not develop fasciculations to the same degree as the nonobese. Because succinylcholine also concomitantly increases the lower esophageal sphincter pressure, the decrease in barrier pressure might be less than anticipated. In a model using pigs with a full stomach and a rapid sequence induction with either propofol or sodium thiopental and succinylcholine, lower esophageal sphincter pressure increased during the fasciculations from 19 ± 4 to 28 ± 5 mm Hg in the propofol-succinylcholine group and from 23 ± 6 to 36 ± 7 mm Hg in the thiopental-succinylcholine group. The lower esophageal sphincter pressure remained elevated after the fasciculations. Similarly, gastric barrier pressure was increased. This increase in barrier pressure begins before fasciculations and remains elevated for the period when intubation would occur, thus protecting against reflux of gastric contents during the typical induction period [59].

Rocuronium is the only nondepolarizing neuromuscular blocking agent with an onset similar to succinylcholine. The side-effect profile is much less problematic than succinylcholine. The duration of action is much longer than succinylcholine, and in patients with an increased risk of difficult airway, rocuronium is not as attractive as succinylcholine during airway difficulties. A recent systematic review by Perry et al [60] compared the intubating conditions of rocuronium with succinylcholine. The authors' conclusions were that succinylcholine creates excellent intubation conditions more reliably than rocuronium and should still be used as a first line muscle relaxant for rapid sequence induction. If an alternative agent is required, rocuronium, when used with propofol, will reliably create excellent intubation conditions and should be used as the second line treatment of choice.

Summary

Patients with obesity and those with sleep apnea syndrome are prone to gastroesophageal reflux. Likewise, both groups demonstrate an increased risk of difficult intubation. Rapid sequence induction remains important in obese and sleep apnea syndrome patients with symptomatic gastroesophageal reflux or other predisposing condition such as diabetes mellitus, pregnancy, emergency surgery, and gastrointestinal conditions. In the case of elective surgery in a fasted patient with no risk factors other than obesity or sleep apnea syndrome, the requirement for rapid sequence induction is debatable. Cricoid pressure is probably efficacious but has not been proven in a randomized, controlled trial to prevent gastric aspiration. The clinician should be aware of the possibility that cricoid pressure will worsen mask ventilation and laryngoscopy and be prepared to loosen or release the pressure if mask ventilation or intubation is compromised. Regular training for the administration of cricoid pressure is indicated. If rapid sequence induction is required, succinylcholine remains the neuromuscular blocking agent of choice if there are no contraindications. Adequate anesthesia and muscle relaxation during induction are vital because coughing or straining during induction is a major risk for pulmonary aspiration.

References

[1] Kluger MT, Short TG. Aspiration during anaesthesia: a review of 133 cases from the Australian Anaesthetic Incident Monitoring Study (AIMS). Anaesthesia 1999;54(1):19–26.

[2] Bond A. Obesity and difficult intubation. Anaesth Intensive Care 1993;21(6):828–30.

[3] Brodsky JB, Lemmens HJ, Brock-Utne JG, et al. Morbid obesity and tracheal intubation. Anesth Analg 2002;94(3):732–6.

[4] Hood DD, Dewan DM. Anesthetic and obstetric outcome in morbidly obese parturients. Anesth 1993;79(6):1210–8.

[5] Rose DK, Cohen MM. The airway: problems and predictions in 18,500 patients. Can J Anaesth 1994;41(5 Pt 1):372–83.

[6] Juvin P, Lavaut E, Dupont H, et al. Difficult tracheal intubation is more common in obese than in lean patients. Anesth Analg 2003;97(2):595–600.

[7] Siyam MA, Benhamou D. Difficult endotracheal intubation in patients with sleep apnea syndrome. Anesth Analg 2002;95(4):1098–102.

[8] Connolly LA. Anaesthetic management of sleep apnoea. J Clin Anesth 1991;3:461–9.

[9] Hillman DR, Platt PR, Eastwood PR. The upper airway during anaesthesia. Br J Anaesth 2003; 91(1):31–9.

[10] Hiremath AS, Hillman DR, James AL, et al. Relationship between difficult tracheal intubation and sleep apnoea. Br J Anaesth 1998;80:606–11.

[11] Reissell E, Orko R, Maunuksela EL, et al. Predictability of difficult laryngoscopy in patients with long-term diabetes mellitus. Anaesthesia 1990;45:1024–7.

[12] Warner MA, Warner ME, Webber JG. Clinical significance of pulmonary aspiration during the perioperative period. Anesthesiology 1993;78:56–62.

[13] Farmery AD, Roe PG. A model to describe the rate of oxyhaemoglobin desaturation during apnoea. Br J Anaesth 1996;76(2):284–91.

[14] Berthoud MC, Peacock JE, Reilly CS. Effectiveness of preoxygenation in morbidly obese patients. Br J Anaesth 1991;67(4):464–6.

[15] Jense HG, Dubin SA, Silverstein PI, et al. Effect of obesity on safe duration of apnea in anesthetized humans. Anesth Analg 1991;72(1):89–93.

[16] Coussa M, Proietti S, Schnyder P, et al. Prevention of atelectasis formation during the induction of general anesthesia in morbidly obese patients. Anesth Analg 2004;98:1491–5.

[17] Allman KG. Effect of cricoid pressure application on airway patency. J Clin Anesth 1995;7(3): 197–9.

[18] Saghaei M, Masoodifar M. The pressor response and airway effects of cricoid pressure during induction of general anesthesia. Anesth Analg 2001;93(3):787–90.

[19] Hartsilver EL, Vanner RG. Airway obstruction with cricoid pressure. Anaesthesia 2000;55:208–11.

[20] Haslam N, Parker L, Duggan JE. Effect of cricoid pressure on the view at laryngoscopy. Anaesthesia 2005;60(1):41–7.

[21] Samsoon G, Young JR. Difficult tracheal intubation: a retrospective study. Anaesthesia 1987; 42:487–90.

[22] Barnardo PD, Jenkins JG. Failed tracheal intubation in obstetrics: a 6-year review in a UK region. Anaesthesia 2000;55:685–94.

[23] Morris J, Cook TM. Rapid sequence induction: a national survey of practice. Anaesthesia 2001; 56:1090–111.

[24] Hood DD, Dewan DM. Anesthetic and obstetric outcome in morbidly obese parturients. Anesthesiology 1993;79(6):1210–8.

[25] Asai T, Barclay K, Power I, et al. Cricoid pressure impeded placement of the laryngeal mask airway. Br J Anaesth 1995;74:521–5.

[26] Aoyama K, Takenaka I, Sata T, et al. Cricoid pressure impedes positioning and ventilation through the laryngeal mask airway. Can J Anaesth 1996;43:1035–40.

[27] Harry RM, Nolan JP. The use of cricoid pressure with the intubating laryngeal mask. Anaesthesia 1999;54:656–9.

[28] Zacchi P, Mearin F, Humbert P, et al. Effect of obesity on gastroesophageal resistance to flow in man. Dig Dis Sci 1991;36(10):1473–80.

[29] Kadar AG, Ing CH, White PF, et al. Anesthesia for electroconvulsive therapy in obese patients. Anesth Analg 2002;94(2):360–1.

[30] Fisher BL, Pennathur A, Mutnick JL, et al. Obesity correlates with gastroesophageal reflux. Dig Dis Sci 1999;44(11):2290–4.

[31] Wajed SA, Streets CG, Bremner CG, et al. Elevated body mass disrupts the barrier to gastro-esophageal reflux. Arch Surg 2001;136:1014–9.

[32] Demeter P, Pap A. The relationship between gastroesophageal reflux disease and obstructive sleep apnea. J Gastroenterol 2004;39(9):815–20.

[33] Morse CA, Quan SF, Mays MZ, et al. Is there a relationship between obstructive sleep apnea and gastroesophageal reflux disease? Clin Gastroenterol Hepatol 2004;2(9):761–8.

[34] Sellick BA. Cricoid pressure to control regurgitation of stomach contents during induction of anaesthesia. Lancet 1961;2:404–6.

[35] Salem MR, Sellick BA, Elam JO. The historical background of cricoid pressure in anesthesia and resuscitation. Anesth Analg 1974;53(2):230–2.

[36] Curry J. Popular observations on apparent death from drowning, suffocation etc. with an account of the means to be employed for recovery. Northampton, UK: T. Dicey and Co; 1792.

[37] Morton HL, Wylie WD. Anaesthetic deaths due to regurgitation or vomiting. Anaesthesia 1951; 6:190–201.

[38] Brimacombe JR, Berry AM. Cricoid pressure. Can J Anaesth 1997;44:414–25.

[39] Ng A, Smith G. Gastroesophageal reflux and aspiration of gastric contents in anesthetic practice. Anesth Analg 2002;93:494–513.

[40] Landsman I. Cricoid pressure: indications and complications. Paediatr Anaesth 2004;14:43–7.

[41] Vanner RG, Pryle BJ. Regurgitation and oesophageal rupture with cricoid pressure: a cadaver study. Anaesthesia 1992;47:732–5.

[42] Vanner RG, O'Dwyer JP, Pryle BJ, et al. Upper oesophageal sphincter pressure and the effect of cricoid pressure. Anaesthesia 1992;47:95–100.

[43] Lawes EG, Campbell I, Mercer D. Inflation pressure, gastric insufflation and rapid sequence induction. Br J Anaesth 1987;59:315–8.

[44] Salem MR, Wong AY, Mani M, et al. Efficacy of cricoid pressure in preventing gastric inflation during bag-mask ventilation in pediatric patients. Anesthesiology 1974;40:96–8.

[45] Moynihan RJ, Brock-Utne JG, Archer JH, et al. The effect of cricoid pressure on preventing gastric insufflation in infants and children. Anesthesiology 1993;78:652–6.

[46] Tournadre J-P, Chassard D, Berrada KR, et al. Cricoid cartilage pressure decreases lower esophageal sphincter tone. Anesth 1997;86(1):7–9.

[47] Garrard A, Campbell AE, Turley A, et al. The effect of mechanically induced cricoid force on lower oesophageal sphincter pressure in anesthetized patients. Anaesthesia 2004;59:435–9.

[48] Tiret L, Desmonts JM, Hatton F, et al. Complications associated with anaesthesia: a prospective survey in France. Can J Anaesth 1986;33:336–44.

[49] Meek T, Gittins N, Duggan JE. Cricoid pressure: knowledge and performance amongst anaes-thetic assistants. Anaesthesia 1999;54:59–62.

[50] Meek T, Vincent A, Duggan JE. Cricoid pressure: can protective force be sustained? Br J Anaesth 1998;80:672–4.

[51] Smith KJ, Dobranowski J, Yip G, et al. Cricoid pressure displaces the esophagus: an obser-vational study using magnetic resonance imaging. Anesthesiology 2003;99:60–4.

[52] Vanner RG. Tolerance of cricoid pressure by conscious volunteers. Int J Obstet Anesth 1992;1: 195–8.

[53] Salem MR, Joseph NJ, Heyman HJ, et al. Cricoid compression is effective in obliterating the esophageal lumen in the presence of a nasogastric tube. Anesthesiology 1985;63(4):443–6.

[54] Haslam N, Syndercombe A, Zimmer CR, et al. Intragastric pressure and its relevance to protec-tive cricoid force. Anaesthesia 2003;58(10):1012–5.

[55] El-Orbany MI, Joseph NJ, Salem MR, et al. The neuromuscular effects and tracheal intubation conditions after small doses of succinylcholine. Anesth Analg 2004;98(6):1680–5.

[56] Naguib M, Samarkandi A, Riad W, et al. Optimal dose of succinylcholine revisited. Anesth 2003;99(5):1045–9.

[57] Sparr HJ. Choice of the muscle relaxant for rapid-sequence induction. Eur J Anaesth 2001; 23(Suppl):S71–6.

[58] Brodsky JB, Foster PE. Succinylcholine and morbid obesity. Obes Surg 2003;13:138–9.

[59] Tournadre JP, Barclay M, Bouletreau P, et al. Lower oesophageal sphincter tone increases after induction of anaesthesia in pigs with full stomach. Can J Anaesth 1998;45:479–82.

[60] Perry J, Lee J, Wells G. Rocuronium versus succinylcholine for rapid sequence induction intubation. Cochrane Database Syst Rev 2003;1:CD 002788.

ELSEVIER
SAUNDERS

Anesthesiology Clin N Am
23 (2005) 565–571

ANESTHESIOLOGY
CLINICS OF
NORTH AMERICA

Index

Note: Page numbers of article titles are in **boldface** type.

A

Ablation, tissue, multilevel radiofrequency, for treatment of obstructive sleep apnea, 531

Adenotonsillectomy, in children, for obstructive sleep apnea treatment, 539–540

Adjustable gastric banding, laparoscopic, management of obesity with, 509–511

Age, as risk factor for obstructive sleep apnea, 412–413

Airway, anatomy of in children, pathophysiology of obstructive sleep apnea and, 536
    assessment, preoperative, in obese patients, 465–466
    difficult, rapid sequence induction and, in patients with obesity and/or obstructive sleep apnea, 552–555

Alcohol consumption, as risk factor for obstructive sleep apnea, 414–415

Anesthesia, in obese patients, **479–486**
    intensity of monitoring required for, 483
    laparoscopy in, 484
    minimizing hypoxia during anesthesia, 484–486
    pharmacokinetics, 479–481
    positioning obese patients for surgery, 481–482
    regional anesthesia in, 482–483
  in patients with obstructive sleep apnea, in children, 542–544
    effects of anesthetic drugs on ventilation responses in, 486–487
    intensity of intraoperative monitoring required, 487
    rational approach to, 488
    technique, 487
  rapid sequence induction in patients with obesity and/or obstructive sleep apnea, **551–564**
    cricoid pressure, 556–560
    induction agent pharmacology, 560–561
    risk of gastroesophageal reflux and pulmonary aspiration, 555–556
    with the difficult airway, 552–555

Apnea-hypopnea index, 407, 446–447

Apnea. See also *Obstructive sleep apnea.*
    definition of, 406–407

Aspiration, pulmonary, risk of, in anesthesia of patients with obesity and/or obstructive sleep apnea, 555–556

Assessment, preoperative.
    See *Preoperative evaluation.*

Atherosclerotic cardiovascular disease, associated with obstructive sleep apnea, 439

B

Banding, gastric, laparoscopic adjustable, management of obesity with, 509–511

Bariatric surgery, 504–520
    choice of surgery, 518–519
    complications, 517–518
    future developments, 517
    indications for, 505
    malabsorptive procedures, 514–516
      biliopancreatic diversion, 514–516
      duodenal switch, 514–516
    overview of surgical procedures, 506–508
    preoperative preparation, 505
    restrictive procedures, 508–514
      laparoscopic adjustable gastric banding, 509–511
      roux-en-Y gastric bypass, 511–514
      vertical gastric banding, 508–509
    simultaneous cholecystectomy with, 519

doi:10.1016/S0889-8537(05)00063-5